FEED ZONE PORTABLES

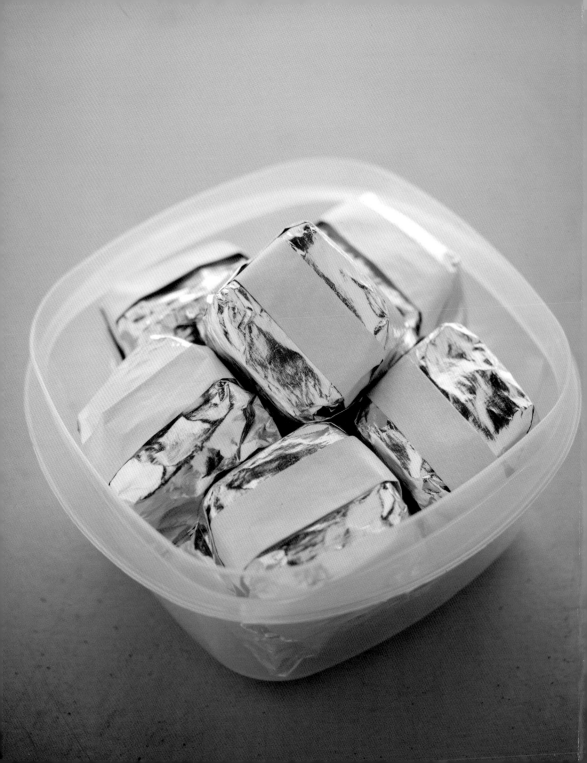

FEED ZONE PORTABLES

A COOKBOOK of ON-THE-GO FOOD for ATHLETES

Biju Thomas & Allen Lim

VELO PRESS

BOULDER, COLORADO

▼ velopress®

3002 Sterling Circle, Suite 100
Boulder, Colorado 80301-2338 USA
(303) 440-0601 ★ Fax (303) 444-6788
E-mail velopress@competitorgroup.com

Distributed in the United States and Canada by Ingram Publisher Services

Library of Congress
Cataloging-in-Publication Data

Thomas, Biju.
    Feed zone portables : a cookbook of on-the-go
    food for athletes / Biju Thomas & Allen Lim.
        pages cm
    Includes index.
    ISBN 978-1-937715-00-7 (hardback)
    1. Athletes--Nutrition. 2. Snack foods. I. Title.
    TX361.A8T56 2013
    641.5'3--dc23
                                2013003073

For information on purchasing VeloPress
books, please call (800) 811-4210 ext. 2138
or visit www.velopress.com.

★

14 15 / 10 9 8 7 6

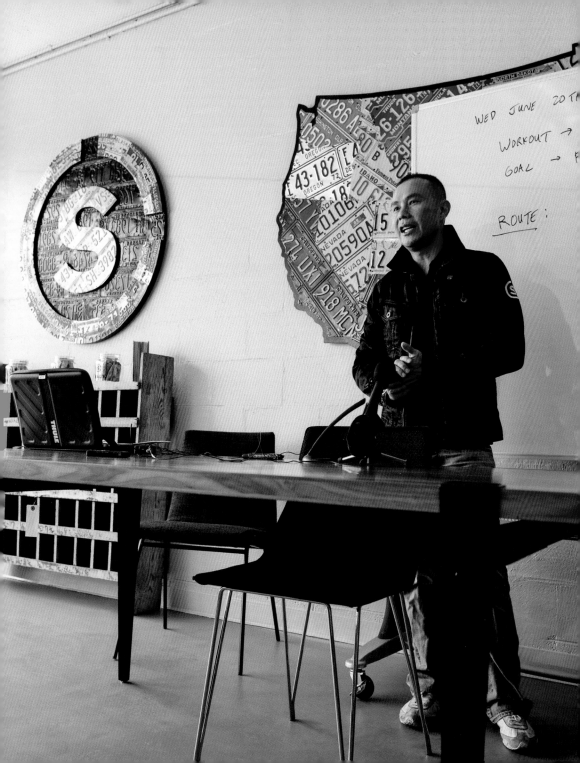

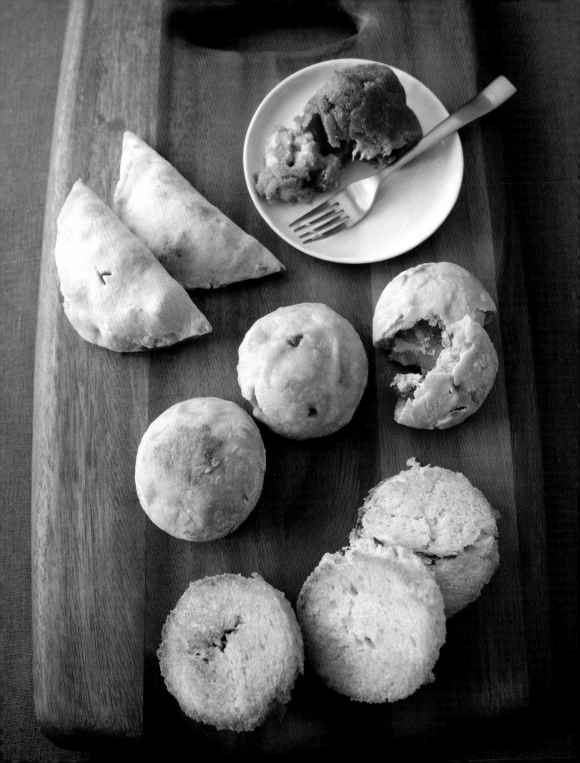

CONTENTS

RICE CAKES

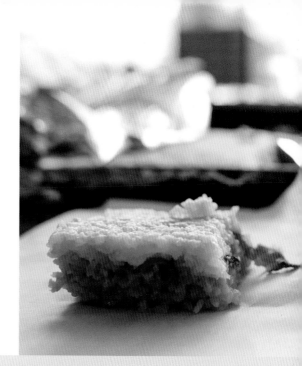

"THESE RECIPES ARE EASY, TASTY, EFFECTIVE, AND **MADE WITH REAL LOVE FOR SPORT AND FOOD.**"

★★★ **GEORGE BENNETT** *RADIOSHACK-LEOPARD-TREK PRO CYCLING TEAM*

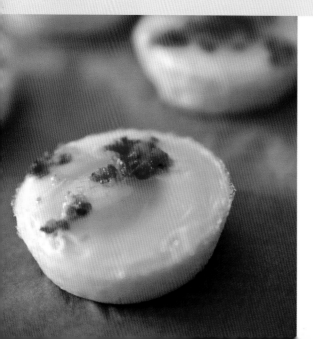

BAKED EGGS

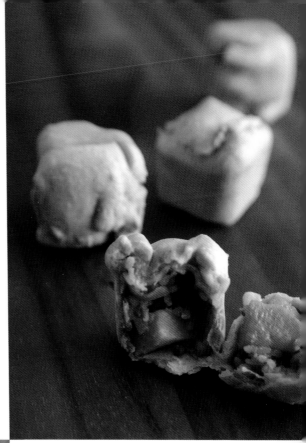

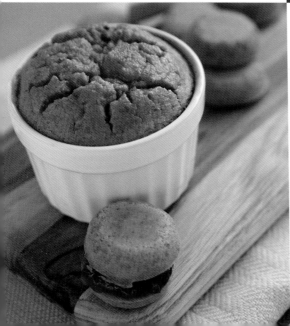

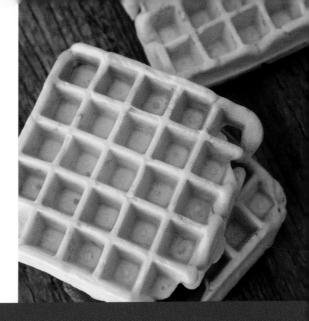

GRIDDLE CAKES, PANCAKES & WAFFLES

"GUT ROT IS NO LONGER AN EXCUSE IN TRIATHLON THANKS TO THE 'REAL FOOD REVOLUTION' CREATED BY ALLEN AND BIJU."

KRISTEN PETERSON *PROFESSIONAL TRIATHLETE*

★ ★ ★

AHA! PORTABLES

TAKE & MAKE

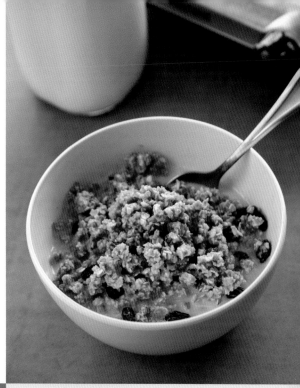

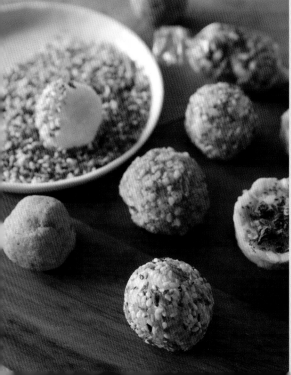

PORTABLES HOW-TO'S

FOREWORDS

I AM A PROFESSIONAL CYCLIST. I burn upward of 5,000 calories on an average day of training and racing. This means there are times when I can eat like a garbage disposal and there are times when I need to hold back, but most importantly, times when I *must* eat. Because I spend so much time on my bike, I'm obligated to eat while keeping said bike in motion. Up until recently, I basically had to force down food. Bars, gels, and mini sandwiches went down the hatch for one sole purpose—energy. While these foods may have done the trick calorically, my level of enjoyment was at an all-time low.

Enter Allen Lim and Biju Thomas. Allen has been a close friend/ training consigliere/psychologist/brain stimulator since 2007. In late 2011 his friend Biju started coming over to my house and graciously hosting dinner parties a couple times a week. I have a new

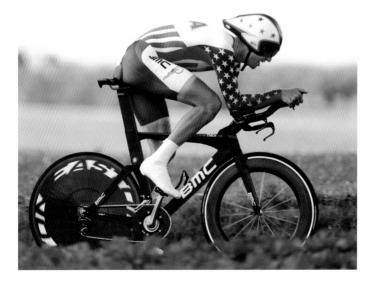

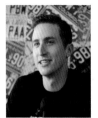

"YOU'RE GOING TO LOVE *FEED ZONE PORTABLES* BECAUSE FROM NOW ON YOU AREN'T GOING TO EAT JUST BECAUSE YOU HAVE TO IN ORDER TO MAKE IT HOME FROM YOUR RIDE."

appreciation for the art of carnitas thanks to this man I call Bij (pronounced *Beeej*). If I could pack Al and Bij into a suitcase and take them everywhere, I would.

My eyes were truly opened to the wonders of *Feed Zone Portables* in the summer of 2012 leading up to the London Olympic Games. Rather than go the traditional route and race my way to fitness over June and July in Europe, I opted to stay in my hometown of Boulder, Colorado, and train very specifically for the Games. This meant I spent a whole lot of hours on the bike, drank many a bottle of Skratch, and had the two best guys in the game preparing food for me. Their support was unparalleled, and I will forever be indebted to them for their commitment to my Olympic dream. When it was all over, returning to normal Euro life proved to be quite difficult. I went from perfectly prepared rice cakes with bacon, almond butter, and maple syrup back to your standard bars and gels, from the greatest chicken fried rice I have ever tasted to two pieces of bread with a slice of cheese and ham.

At least I can control what I put into my body at home, which is why a book like this is invaluable. Whether you're like me or just a casual Sunday cyclist, you're going to love *Feed Zone Portables* because from now on you aren't going to eat just because you have to in order to make it home from your ride. You will reach into your back pocket for a Feed Zone portable and feel like a kid with a candy bar. You will be rewarding your body with the goodness within these pages. Don't be surprised if you ride longer and harder than ever before.

TAYLOR PHINNEY
2-TIME OLYMPIAN
PROFESSIONAL CYCLIST, BMC RACING TEAM

EATING FOR FUEL had been a struggle for me throughout my cycling career. I spent my summers road racing and my winters racing cyclo-cross, so it seemed as though I was always racing, traveling, or resting. Constantly trying to keep my energy level up at the right times and avoid food at the wrong times was consuming too much time and energy. It was exhausting.

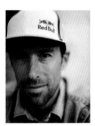

"I BELIEVE THAT NOT KNOWING WHAT TO EAT AND WHEN TO EAT IT CAN BE AS DETRIMENTAL TO PERFORMANCE AS SHIRKING YOUR TRAINING."

Like a lot of other young cyclists, I fell victim to poor habits and misinformation. I found myself cutting out this or eating more of that in hopes of going faster. I eventually learned that virtually anything "worked" for a time. But adapting my lifestyle and food choices to match my true needs was really the only way to make a lasting impact on my performance.

I met Biju and Allen a few years ago at the Ride on Washington, where they were tasked with feeding riders and staff. I poked my head into the trailer the first morning at around 5:30 a.m. Biju was knee-deep in oatmeal, while Allen was shuttling food in and out and trying to get the coffee maker working. It was controlled chaos, but it was clear they were going to turn out some tasty grub. One bite showed me a lot of what I was missing.

Eating real, flavorful, and simple food was a revelation. I began eating more energy-dense foods when I needed them and lighter meals with more fiber when I was resting or traveling. Instead of just eating something I considered healthy before a ride—like cereal and yogurt—I was eating oatmeal with eggs on top (and maple syrup, my all-time favorite). Instead of finishing a ride and eating a tuna fish sandwich an hour later, I was pulling warm rice out of the cooker and eating while still in my cycling shorts.

Being around Allen and Biju began to ground me and my diet. Over the summer months, I spent long hours riding with my training partners in Boulder and plowing through plate after plate of rice and eggs. After tough workouts where we pushed ourselves to the limit over and over, it was liberating to be rid of any apprehension about what or how much to eat. It meant we had enough energy left over to give each other shit, or maybe even start thinking about the next workout.

Good food may only be a portion of what it takes to ride professionally, but to me it has been truly life changing. I believe that not knowing what to eat and when to eat it can be as detrimental to performance as shirking your training. Now that my nutrition is dialed in, I can focus on the other important aspects of training and racing. I hope you too can find a new relationship with eating through Biju and Allen's delicious creations.

TIM JOHNSON
CANNONDALE P/B
CYCLOCROSSWORLD.COM

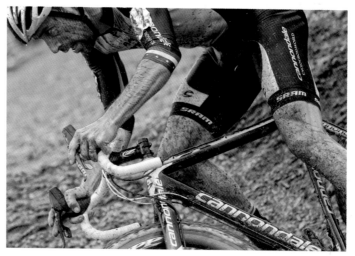

PREFACE

SINCE THE LAUNCH OF *THE FEED ZONE COOKBOOK*, Chef Biju and I have received a lot of questions from athletes around what to eat while exercising, traveling, or on the go. The "Portables" section of our first cookbook presented a number of recipes for real food that can be eaten during activity, and it started a conversation about the rationale and science behind what to eat when training and competing.

Attempting to answer any question about science or theory is only part of the equation when it comes to the evolving discussion around nutrition and performance. The practice of making real food is not always easy, especially when our lives are busy and stressful. But when all is said and done, we still need and want healthy, fresh, and simple portable foods to keep us fueled and nourished when we're on the move.

It's our hope that *Feed Zone Portables* will take your practice a step further by giving you some of the science behind eating when heart rates are higher than normally found at the dinner table and providing a greater variety of easy-to-follow, real-food portable recipes and ideas for the times when you're away from the table.

ALLEN LIM

INTRODUCTION

An entire pre-packaged sports nutrition industry has evolved to provide athletes and even nonathletes with portable foods that run the gamut from energy bars to gooey gels. Because so many of these products are designed with the intent of optimizing exercise performance, it's easy to become swayed by the convenience and promise of these products rather than the ingredients or real-world results they provide. We've all bought into the ease of pre-packaged foods when literally on the "run" even if we don't necessarily enjoy them, or worse, even when they make us feel bad. Is it science we're buying? Convenience? Or a marketing myth? More important, are energy bars and engineered sports nutrition actually better for us than eating real food?

I've worked with very few athletes who could eat pre-packaged foods all day when training or competing. They would often complain that they just couldn't stomach the bars, blocks, and gels given to them (ironically, these often were the same products they helped to market). Instead, many of these athletes would pack real-food snacks to take with them on long days of training—little sandwiches, fresh pastries, and even leftover pizza. They turned to real food not because of some claim on the label but because through their own trial and error, they learned it made them feel better. It was not a scientific study that led me to work with Chef Biju to find better solutions to the conventional sports nutrition being sold. It was the athletes themselves—their experiences and feedback—that inspired me to take the extra time to start cooking from scratch.

Anecdotally, I can definitively say that real food works—the athletes Chef Biju and I consulted with felt better and performed better when they ate freshly prepared food instead of pre-packaged bars. While that may be common sense, we can all agree that making real food is often inconvenient. In fact, every morning I made fresh portable foods at the Tour de France, I cursed the process. As much as I love food and love to cook, prepping food for competitive events is not some Zen-like activity that helps me achieve a state of perfection or grace. Like most people, I don't normally have the time for it even

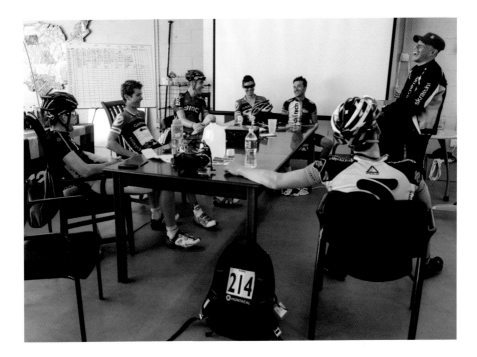

when I am motivated to make the extra effort. But I knew how much it helped the athletes to perform. If it weren't for that simple fact, I would never have spent the time to make fresh portable food when it really mattered. If pre-packaged food worked better, I would have been the first person to use it exclusively.

At the 2012 Olympic Games in London, I went to great lengths to find the right ingredients for preparing fresh ride food for members of the US Olympic cycling team, at times putting myself at extreme physical risk to get the job done. Team USA was staying outside of the city to avoid the throngs of tourists, so I

rented a little scooter (from what seemed like a group of amiable Russian mobsters) to pick up some groceries from the best organic markets in London. I strapped a huge duffle bag to my back, put on my helmet and my best motor-pacing boots, and began the hour-long jaunt into London. Zipping in and out of some of the craziest traffic I've ever experienced on what was the wrong side of the road for me, while navigating old-school style with a paper map and street signs, it took me most of the jaw-clenching afternoon to hit all the markets on my list. With my duffle bag heavy with groceries and cooking supplies, I took a moment to get my bearings in the heart of London. I noticed some tourists pointing up at a tower and looked up only to realize that a military sniper on top had his rifle aimed right at me. I think he sensed the avocado bombs ready to explode in my bag. Taking the advice of Winston Churchill, I kept calm, gave the sniper a shaky wave, and carried on.

doing, it just takes a little practice and planning. I will concede that when you are traveling or short on time, pre-packaged energy bars and snacks are often unavoidable, but *easy* or *convenient* does not mean *better*. There's nothing easy about being an athlete. Hard work and discipline are aspects of sport and athleticism that

Hard work and discipline are aspects of sport and athleticism that we naturally accept and are drawn to. Extending that idea to include something as important as nutrition is critical if you want the gains associated with that effort or if you just can't stomach the pre-packaged options.

Luckily, I didn't get my head blown off, and in the end the effort was totally worth it. I made fresh portables for the riders to train with, and on the morning of the Olympic road race I had the honor of wrapping a massive number of rice cakes with assistance from the legendary Davis Phinney. His son, Taylor, would go on to finish fourth in both the road race and time trial events—a heart-breaking but extraordinary set of performances for a twenty-two-year-old. On the morning of the Olympic time trial, I got a special request from Kristin Armstrong for Biju's Oatmeal, which I prepped in the hotel's kitchen. Later that afternoon, Kristin went on to win her second gold medal, fueled by a simple bowl of oatmeal, which I now affectionately refer to as Gold Medal Oatmeal.

See Portable Oatmeal on p. 232

While the Olympics merit an extreme effort, cooking real food doesn't have to be an all-out chore. Like most things worth

we naturally accept and are drawn to. Extending that idea to include something as important as our nutrition is critical if you want the gains associated with that effort or, if like many athletes, you just can't stomach or simply don't like the pre-packaged options.

There will always be a market for pre-packaged foods, and the reality is that I will not always be able to avoid them myself. But, the more I've thought about why the athletes I work with prefer real food, the more I've realized that there are a lot of misnomers—if not complete myths—about the pre-packaged foods sold to us. Beginning with basic notions about what we actually need to eat or drink during exercise and extending to a lack of knowledge about how our gastrointestinal tract works to digest and process the calories we consume—there are misconceptions that deserve a closer look.

FIRST ASK THIS › DO YOU REALLY NEED TO EAT THAT?

If you've ever run out of fuel while exercising and "bonked" or "hit the wall," then you know how important eating early and often is to performance. This is why I am constantly preaching the importance of eating and drinking during long-term endurance exercise. However, once we take a look at the numbers I think you'll agree that in many situations we are better served not eating anything when we're exercising.

Energy-rich foods are fantastic if you're running, riding, or hiking for long periods of time, but they're not always necessary and are potentially harmful if you eat regular meals, spend a lot of your day sitting, and are exercising or competing for less than two hours. It's all too easy to overestimate the calories we burn during exercise and underestimate the calories we actually consume. So before you go tearing open a bunch of sports bars or cooking up any of the recipes in this book, figure out how much you actually need to eat when you are exercising. I'll be the first to tell you to put down that rice cake or sports drink if you aren't working and sweating for it.

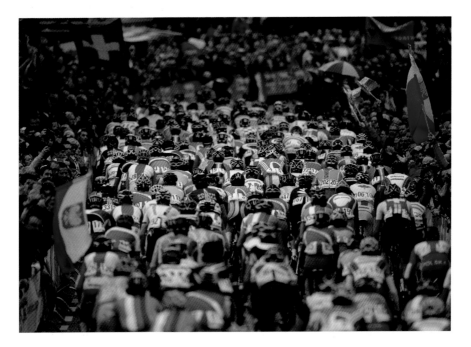

CALCULATING CALORIE DEFICITS

Here's an overview of figuring out how many calories you need to eat during exercise:

1 Figure out how many calories you are burning.

The fitter you are, the harder you are working; the less efficient you are, and the bigger you are, the more calories you'll be burning.

As a point of reference, the best athletes in the world are hard-pressed to burn more than 1,000 Calories per hour for more than 3 hours.

2 Figure out how many of the calories you are burning are coming from fat versus carbohydrate.

We use primarily fat and carbohydrate during exercise and almost no protein except under extreme situations. At high exercise intensities we burn mostly carbohydrate, and at low intensities we burn mostly fat.

At 50% of maximal aerobic capacity, about 45–55% of calories come from fat; at 75% of max this drops to about 10–30%; and at max (100%), none of our calories come from fat.

3 Figure out how many carbohydrate calories you have stored as glycogen.

Because fat stores are ample, it's almost impossible to run out of it during exercise. But glycogen stores are limited, and once it's gone, it's impossible to maintain high intensity, difficult to maintain your blood sugar (which is critical for fueling your brain and nervous system), and harder to burn fat, all of which can cause fatigue.

On a moderate-carbohydrate diet (40–50% of total intake) an athlete will have about 1,000 Calories available for lower body exercise, and on a high-carbohydrate diet (60–70% of total intake) those stores can double to about 2,000 Calories.

4 Subtract the calories burned from the total calories coming from fat and the total calories of stored glycogen to calculate what you need to eat.

For example, let's say that you burn 2,000 Calories over a 3-hour bike ride and that 500 of those calories come from fat and 1,000 come from stored glycogen. In this scenario, subtracting 2,000 Calories from 1,500 Calories (total calories from fat and carbohydrates) gives a 500 Calorie deficit.

$$
\begin{aligned}
&- 2000 \text{ Calories burned} \\
&+ 500 \text{ Calories from fat} \\
&+ 1000 \text{ Calories stored as glycogen} \\
\hline
& 500 \text{ Calorie carbohydrate deficit}
\end{aligned}
$$

If there's a deficit, *eat*. If there's not, don't eat.

As a general rule of thumb, **for activities lasting more than 2 hours,** if you **eat at least half the calories you burn each hour,** you'll almost always be consuming an adequate number of calories to keep you going.

To dive into the specific details, read on.

CALCULATING THE CALORIES BURNED DURING EXERCISE

The energy, or calories, you burn during exercise primarily depends on your size or body weight, your fitness, your efficiency, and the duration of your exercise. If you're really fit, have a lot of mass, and are going really hard and long, you'll use many more calories than someone who is unfit, lighter, going easy, and only out for a short effort.

For perspective on how many calories are burned during exercise, I'll use the example of cycling at different speeds (mph) and power outputs (watts), and running at different speeds (mph) and paces (minutes per mile).

To accurately estimate the Calories, or kcals, burned per hour while cycling, we need to know a few things. The first is the intensity, which is reflected in the power output and also, depending upon the terrain, the speed. The second is the duration of the ride—in this case one hour. Finally, we need to know a person's efficiency on the bicycle. For reference, the calories burned

TABLE 1› CYCLING: Estimating Calories Burned per Hour

| POWER | SPEED | KJ | CORRECTION FACTOR (CF × kilojoules = kcals) AND % EFFICIENCY | | | | | | |
| | | | 1.19 | 1.14 | 1.09 | 1.04 | 1.00 | 0.96 | 0.92 |
watts	mph	per hr.	20%	21%	22%	23%	24%	25%	26%
400	25.2	1,440	1,720	1,638	1,564	1,496	1,433	1,376	1,323
350	24.1	1,260	1,505	1,433	1,368	1,309	1,254	1,204	1,158
300	22.8	1,080	1,290	1,229	1,173	1,122	1,075	1,032	992
275	22.0	990	1,183	1,126	1,075	1,028	985	946	910
250	21.3	900	1,075	1,024	977	935	896	860	827
225	20.5	810	968	921	880	841	806	774	744
200	19.6	720	860	819	782	748	717	688	662
175	18.7	630	753	717	684	654	627	602	579
150	17.6	540	645	614	586	561	538	516	496
125	16.4	450	538	512	489	467	448	430	413
100	15.1	360	430	410	391	374	358	344	331
75	13.4	270	323	307	293	280	269	258	248
50	11.3	180	215	205	195	187	179	172	165

Calories burned per hour while cycling at different power outputs or speeds on a flat road at a range of gross mechanical efficiencies. At 200 watts or 19.6 mph and a gross mechanical efficiency of 22 percent, a person burns about 782 Calories per hour. Correction factors are also given to convert kilojoules (kJ) of work to calories. Multiply kilojoules by the correction factor associated with a particular gross mechanical efficiency to obtain calories.

per hour while cycling on a flat road have been calculated for different power outputs and speeds over a range of efficiencies and are listed in Table 1. Most people are only 22 percent efficient (see Efficiency: How Far Will a Calorie Take You? page 8).

Table 2 estimates the calories burned per hour while running on flat terrain at different speeds and paces listed for a range of body weights. These estimates are based on standard equations for estimating the oxygen needed per kilogram of body weight developed by the American College of Sports Medicine. The amount of oxygen we consume is directly proportional to the calories we burn.

Ultimately, these references are meant to give you a better sense of the calories you might burn for a given task. For example, even if you don't run regularly, you might be able to guess the fastest you can run a mile, then based on your body weight you can get a sense of how many calories you would burn if

TABLE 2› RUNNING/WALKING: Estimating Calories Burned per Hour

SPEED		BODY WEIGHT									
min. per mile	mph	50 kg	55 kg	60 kg	65 kg	70 kg	75 kg	80 kg	85 kg	90 kg	100 kg
		110 lbs.	121 lbs.	132 lbs.	143 lbs.	154 lbs.	165 lbs.	176 lbs.	187 lbs.	198 lbs.	220 lbs.
4:00	15.0	1,212	1,333	1,454	1,575	1,696	1,818	1,939	2,060	2,181	2,423
5:00	12.0	979	1,077	1,175	1,273	1,371	1,469	1,567	1,665	1,763	1,959
6:00	10.0	825	907	990	1,072	1,154	1,237	1,319	1,402	1,484	1,649
7:00	8.6	714	785	857	928	1,000	1,071	1,142	1,214	1,285	1,428
8:00	7.5	631	694	757	820	883	947	1,010	1,073	1,136	1,262
9:00	6.7	567	623	680	736	793	850	906	963	1,020	1,133
10:00	6.0	515	566	618	669	721	772	824	875	927	1,030
11:00	5.5	473	520	567	614	662	709	756	804	851	945
12:00	5.0	437	481	525	569	612	656	700	744	787	875
14:00	4.3	216	238	260	281	303	324	346	368	389	433
16:00	3.8	196	215	235	254	274	293	313	332	352	391
18:00	3.3	179	197	215	233	251	269	287	305	323	359
20:00	3.0	167	183	200	216	233	250	266	283	300	333

Calories burned per hour at different running and walking speeds over level terrain. For running oxygen consumption per kilogram of body weight per minute (VO_2 ml·kg^{-1}·min^{-1}) is calculated as 0.2 × velocity in meters per second + 3.5. For walking (speed ‹ 5 mph), oxygen consumption per kilogram of body weight per minute is calculated as 0.1 × velocity in meters per second + 3.5. Calories are then calculated based on body weight and by assuming that 4.8 Calories are burned per liter of oxygen consumed. At a 6-minute per mile pace or 10 mph and a body weight of 70 kg (154 lb.), a person burns about 1,154 Calories per hour.

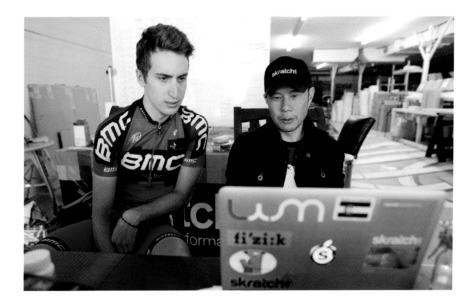

EFFICIENCY: HOW FAR WILL A CALORIE TAKE YOU?

Efficiency describes the relationship between how many calories we burn and how many of those calories actually get converted to real work. As an example, if you are 22 percent efficient and you burn 100 Calories, only 22 Calories actually go into the pedals to make the bicycle move. The other 78 Calories get wasted as heat. While there is likely a big genetic component to efficiency, generally speaking, someone who has just finished the Tour de France is going to be a lot more efficient than someone who just started riding a bicycle. This same idea may also be true for other sports—given the right genetic attributes, experience and practice may lead to improved efficiency.

If you'd like to know how efficient you are, it's relatively easy to find out in any exercise physiology laboratory that can measure oxygen consumption and power output. But if you don't want the hassle of going to the lab, you might be able to make an educated guess as to how efficient you are. If you tend to need more food for a given activity compared to people of similar size and weight, you're probably less efficient. Efficient athletes can essentially do more work with less food because less of what they consume is lost as heat, and this translates to better gas mileage. While this is great for performance, the drawback is that when efficient athletes aren't working out a lot, many often have a hard time keeping excess fat off.

you tried to keep that up for an hour. If anything, use the references to establish a high bar for the maximum number of calories you can burn for your current fitness. Practically speaking, our sense of feel is a valuable tool, and if you rate your effort level on a simple 1 to 10 scale with your 10 or max effort calibrated relative to that high bar, you can better guess your caloric expenditure for submaximal efforts based on feel.

As an example, if running a seven-minute mile is an all-out or "10" level effort for you and you weigh 165 pounds, you'd burn roughly 1,071 Calories if you kept that pace up for an hour. Knowing that's probably not possible, if you went out for an hour run at half that level of effort, it's probably fair to guess that you burned about 500 Calories, or half the max.

The point of all of this is that you have to be really fit to burn a lot of calories when exercising. Most of us would be hard pressed to burn more than 1,000 Calories during an hour of exercise. In fact, even actually need to eat depends on the calories you burn minus the energy you have stored in your body.

FUEL STORES: WHERE FAT IS PLENTIFUL & GLYCOGEN IS NOT

Our two primary forms of energy storage are the fat stored in adipose tissue and the carbohydrate stored as glycogen in muscles and the liver. Even very lean athletes have plenty of fat stores, so fat is not thought of as a rate-limiting fuel source. As an example, at 3,500 Calories per pound of fat, a person weighing 150 pounds with just 10 percent body fat has 15 pounds of stored fat, which is the equivalent of 52,500 Calories. If we figure it takes 100 Calories to walk a mile using fat, that person could theoretically walk 525 miles before he or she ran out of energy. But it's not quite so simple.

Glycogen is the limiting factor; when it's depleted it can severely limit our exercise capacity. This is because our nervous system and brain rely solely on glucose—the most basic unit of carbohydrate in the

Outside of our actual energy expenditure, the amount of glycogen we have stored in working muscle is one of the biggest determinants of what we need to eat. ... The more glycogen we can store, the better off we'll be.

at events like the Tour de France, it's rare to see most riders burn more than 1,000 Calories, and they weigh in at an average of 70 kg (154 lb.).

Once you have a sense of how many calories you might be using, how much you body. When glycogen stores are low and exercise intensity is high, we risk becoming hypoglycemic or having low blood sugar, which can bring us to a standstill. In addition, we need a little bit of carbohydrate to keep some of the metabolic pathways responsible for fat utilization functioning. In many ways, fat is like the wax in a candle while carbohydrate is like the wick. Even if we have plenty of fat or wax, we need a little bit of carbohydrate as a wick to keep the fat or wax burning. Ultimately, outside of our actual energy expenditure, the amount of glycogen we have stored in working muscle is one of the biggest determinants of what we need to eat. Because it's not always possible to get in enough calories while exercising, the more glycogen we can store, the better off we'll be.

TABLE 3› GLYCOGEN: Estimating Calories Available for Lower-Leg Exercise

BODY FAT (%)	TOTAL BODY WEIGHT									
	50 kg 110 lbs.	55 kg 121 lbs.	60 kg 132 lbs.	65 kg 143 lbs.	70 kg 154 lbs.	75 kg 165 lbs.	80 kg 176 lbs.	85 kg 187 lbs.	90 kg 198 lbs.	95 kg 209 lbs.
5.0%	973	1,070	1,167	1,265	1,362	1,459	1,556	1,654	1,751	1,848
7.5%	947	1,042	1,137	1,231	1,326	1,421	1,516	1,610	1,705	1,800
10.0%	922	1,014	1,106	1,198	1,290	1,382	1,475	1,567	1,659	1,751
12.5%	896	986	1,075	1,165	1,254	1,344	1,434	1,523	1,613	1,702
15.0%	870	957	1,044	1,132	1,219	1,306	1,393	1,480	1,567	1,654
17.5%	845	929	1,014	1,098	1,183	1,267	1,352	1,436	1,521	1,605
20.0%	819	901	983	1,065	1,147	1,229	1,311	1,393	1,475	1,556
22.5%	794	873	952	1,032	1,111	1,190	1,270	1,349	1,428	1,508
25.0%	768	845	922	998	1,075	1,152	1,229	1,306	1,382	1,459
5.0%	1,702	1,873	2,043	2,213	2,383	2,554	2,724	2,894	3,064	3,235
7.5%	1,658	1,823	1,989	2,155	2,321	2,486	2,652	2,818	2,984	3,149
10.0%	1,613	1,774	1,935	2,097	2,258	2,419	2,580	2,742	2,903	3,064
12.5%	1,568	1,725	1,882	2,038	2,195	2,352	2,509	2,666	2,822	2,979
15.0%	1,523	1,676	1,828	1,980	2,132	2,285	2,437	2,589	2,742	2,894
17.5%	1,478	1,626	1,774	1,922	2,070	2,218	2,365	2,513	2,661	2,809
20.0%	1,434	1,577	1,720	1,864	2,007	2,150	2,294	2,437	2,580	2,724
22.5%	1,389	1,528	1,667	1,805	1,944	2,083	2,222	2,361	2,500	2,639
25.0%	1,344	1,478	1,613	1,747	1,882	2,016	2,150	2,285	2,419	2,554

Moderate-carb diet brackets rows 5.0%–25.0% (first group). *High-carb diet* brackets rows 5.0%–25.0% (second group).

An estimate of the total calories available for lower-leg exercise from stored muscle glycogen on a moderate-carbohydrate diet (40–50 percent), and on a high-carbohydrate diet (60–75 percent), assuming lower-leg mass equals 32 percent of body weight. This table does not reflect glycogen stored in the liver—a total that may range from 60 to 80 grams of carbohydrate, or 240 to 360 additional Calories on a moderate-carbohydrate diet, or from 100 to 120 grams of carbohydrate, or 400 to 480 additional Calories on a high-carbohydrate diet.

As we become more fit, we're able to use more fat at a given exercise intensity, which allows us to spare our precious glycogen stores.

The amount of glycogen we have stored in our bodies can vary greatly and is affected by a number of factors, particularly how much carbohydrate we eat, how active we are, and our extent of lean muscle mass. As a simple rule of thumb, about 1 or 2 percent of the weight in lean muscle is glycogen. On a moderate-carbohydrate diet there can be anywhere from 15 to 17 grams of carbohydrate per kilogram of muscle, or 60–68 Calories. On a high-carbohydrate diet, the amount of carbohydrate stored in muscle can be almost double, equivalent to 100–120 Calories.

ESTIMATING STORED GLYCOGEN

DIET	% CARBS	CARB/KG MUSCLE	CALORIES*
Moderate-Carb	40–50%	15–17 g	60–68
High-Carb	60–70%	25–30 g	100–120

*Calculated at 4 Calories per gram of carbohydrate

While it may be simple to think that the total glycogen stored in the body can be calculated by simply multiplying the figures above by one's body weight or lean muscle mass, calculating the available glycogen for a given activity is a little more complex. This is because a particular muscle can only access the glycogen inside of it, not the glycogen in other muscles. Your quads, for example, can't tap into the glycogen stored in your biceps.

Available glycogen is essentially limited to whatever is stored in the muscle doing the actual work (i.e., working muscle). For a person who weighs 70 kg (154 lb.) and has 10 percent body fat, about 630 grams of glycogen are stored in muscle (1 percent of 63 kg of lean mass). During lower-leg exercise like cycling or running, however, only about 30–35 percent of the total muscle mass is being used, so the actual glycogen available for cycling in this example is closer to 221 grams (at 35 percent). At 4 Calories per gram of carbohydrate, the total stored carbohydrate calories available for lower-leg exercise is about 882 Calories. In addition to glycogen stored in muscle, about 80 to 120 grams of glycogen can be stored in the liver, which can account for an additional 320 to 480 Calories available to help maintain blood sugar and to fuel any muscle.

To simplify things, I've provided an estimation of available calories stored as glycogen for lower-leg exercise for both moderate-carbohydrate and high-carbohydrate diets. Table 3 estimates the total calories available from glycogen based upon body weight, body fat percentage, and assuming an average lower-leg mass equal to 32 percent of total body weight. This average for lower-leg mass was obtained from hundreds of scans of cyclists I've worked with using a low-energy X-ray that measures body composition.

The amount of glycogen stored in muscle is finite, so whether we tap into these stores depends not only on the carbohydrate that we might eat during exercise but also (and primarily) on the percentage of fat versus carbohydrate used while exercising. Generally speaking, more fat is used at lower relative exercise intensities while more carbohydrate is used at higher relative exercise intensities. As we become more fit, we're able to use more fat at a given exercise intensity, which allows us to spare our precious glycogen stores.

FUEL FROM CARBOHYDRATE AND FAT RELATIVE TO INTENSITY

PERCENTAGE OF MAX	FUEL FROM CARBOHYDRATE	FUEL FROM FAT
25%	~20–30%	~70–80%
50%	~45–55%	~55–45%
75%	~70–90%	~10–30%
100%	100%	–

Note: Fuel depends on intensity, or the percentage of one's maximal aerobic capacity.

While you may wonder if protein is used during exercise, the simple answer is rarely—only in extremely stressful situations when carbohydrate stores are nearly depleted and the need to maintain blood sugar levels is at a premium. If you've ever reached a point during long-term exercise where you begin to smell ammonia in your sweat or urine, then you've actually pushed yourself to a point where you're breaking down protein and using it as a fuel source. Hitting this "ammonia" threshold is extremely rare and almost never occurs if a person is eating enough carbohydrate. To be able to push yourself to this point requires an incredible level of fitness and drive—most people will quit before they reach this point. Though protein is important to help maintain and build muscle mass and is critical for proper recovery and as part of a well-balanced diet, except in extreme situations it is not a significant or important fuel source during exercise.

CALCULATING WHAT WE ACTUALLY NEED TO EAT

Putting it all together, the amount we need to eat depends on the calories we are burning and whether we have the energy stores, primarily in the form of glycogen, to meet that demand. If we have enough fat and glycogen on board to meet the caloric demand for a given duration and intensity, then we don't have to worry about eating.

However, when your exercise intensity is high and prolonged, making sure you eat enough is critical. Let's assume that you are fit enough to burn 2,000 Calories over two hours and that at this intensity and duration, 95 percent of your calories will come from carbohydrate. Let's also assume that there are only 1,500 Calories of glycogen available.

–2000 Calories burned over 2 hours
+100 Calories from fat (5%)
+1500 Calories from glycogen
───────────────────────────
400 Calorie carbohydrate deficit

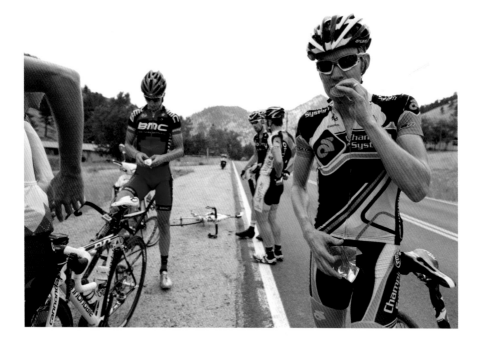

If we do the math, first factoring in your energy stores, there are just 400 Calories, or 100 grams of carbohydrate, that need to be eaten over the course of the effort to maintain performance.

It may not seem like a lot compared to the calories burned, but eating 400 Calories (the equivalent of two energy bars) over the course of two hours is not trivial, especially when you are going hard. Timing your calories is also important. You must keep the carbohydrate tank full if you want to maintain high-intensity exercise. In fact, if you didn't eat something prior to beginning exercise, at a high, real-time burn rate you might find yourself running on fumes sooner than you think. While eating fat or protein may spare some carbohydrate, at high intensities no amount of extra fat or protein is going to make up for carbohydrate.

As the effort gets longer, intensity naturally drops. This is the intensity you are likely to maintain over the course of riding a century (100 miles) and when running a marathon (26.2 miles). Given the lower intensity, it would be more likely that 75 percent of the energy burned comes from carbohydrate and 25 percent comes from fat.

Table 4 lists a range of times for a 70-kg (154-lb.) cyclist to ride a windless, flat century at different speeds and estimated power outputs. Assuming our cyclist is 21 percent efficient, we can estimate the number of calories he will burn per minute, per hour, and the total calories required. Let's again count on glycogen in active muscle supplying 1,500 Calories of carbohydrate. Adding this to the calories supplied from fat, we can find out how much our cyclist will need to eat.

$$-3919 \text{ Calories burned over } 5.5 \text{ hours}$$
$$+980 \text{ Calories from fat } (25\%)$$
$$+1500 \text{ Calories from glycogen}$$
$$\overline{1439 \text{ Calorie carbohydrate deficit}}$$

Once we account for the energy stores, 1,439 additional Calories from carbohydrate will be needed over the course of the 5.5 hours to maintain the performance.

Because the effort is not as intense, our cyclist should be able to keep up with this demand (262 Calories per hour).

It would be extraordinarily difficult to ride a century in under 4:30 without drafting, a time trial bicycle, or a tucked position. For most of us, these calculations would be unsustainable for the full duration, though for shorter durations the calculations for these intensities are still relevant.

Similarly, Table 5 lists a range of times for a 70-kg (154-lb.) athlete to run a marathon on a flat course. The athlete's estimated oxygen consumption per kilogram of body weight is calculated based on the pace per mile. The calories expended per minute, per hour, and the total calories

TABLE 4› **RIDING A CENTURY: Estimating Carbohydrate Deficits**

TIME hrs:min.	SPEED mph	POWER watts	CALORIES per min.	CALORIES per hr.	TOTAL CAL.	CALORIES FROM Stored Fat	CALORIES FROM Carbs	CARB CAL. NEEDED TO EAT Total	CARB CAL. NEEDED TO EAT per hr.
6:30	15.4	108	8	464	3,014	754	2,261	761	117
6:00	16.7	133	9	568	3,410	853	2,558	1,058	176
5:30	18.2	166	12	713	3,919	980	2,939	1,439	262
5:10	19.4	196	14	841	4,343	1,086	3,258	1,758	340
4:50	20.7	235	17	1,005	4,859	1,215	3,644	2,144	444
4:30	22.2	285	20	1,220	5,492	1,373	4,119	2,619	582
4:10	23.8	343	24	1,469	6,121	1,530	4,590	3,090	742

Without changing your bike drafting position, this would be very difficult.

An estimate of the calories needed to ride a century at different speeds on a flat and windless course without draft for a 70-kg (154-lb.) person riding in an upright position. The total calories burned and estimate of calories from fat versus carbohydrate are calculated assuming that 75 percent of the calories burned are derived from carbohydrate. Based on an estimated 1,500 Calories of stored glycogen in active muscle (i.e., muscles used for pedaling), the total carbohydrate that must be consumed is estimated by subtracting calories from glycogen.

burned are derived from the estimated oxygen consumption for each speed. Given the distance of the effort, we'll again assume that 75 percent of the calories are derived from carbohydrate and that 1,500 Calories are available from stored glycogen to calculate the calories derived from carbohydrate versus fat and also to estimate the total carbohydrate needed to perform each time.

My goal in walking you through all of these calculations and hypothetical situations is to give you a better perspective on the calories that you might actually use when exercising. The numbers aren't precise, and there are many variables at play, but this much is true:

Most of us don't need to eat more than **400 Calories per hour** for events lasting 2–6 hours.

For events lasting longer than 2–3 hours, if you make it your goal to **replace half of the calories you burn per hour,** you will almost always be eating more than enough to sustain the effort.

Although not eating enough can clearly be detrimental to one's performance, the reality is that eating more won't make up for a lack of fitness. Putting more fuel in a car doesn't make the engine bigger; in fact, all it does is spill over into the main compartments and create a ticking time bomb.

TABLE 5› RUNNING A MARATHON: Estimating Carbohydrate Deficits

TIME hrs:min.	PACE min. per mile	VO₂ ml/kg/ min.	CALORIES per min.	CALORIES per hr.	TOTAL CAL.	CALORIES FROM Stored Fat	CALORIES FROM Carbs	CARB CAL. NEEDED TO EAT Total	CARB CAL. NEEDED TO EAT per hr.
6:30	14:53	14	5	301	1,957	489	1,468	-32	-5
5:30	12:36	16	6	342	1,883	471	1,412	-88	-16
4:30	10:18	35	12	731	3,289	822	2,467	967	215
3:30	8:01	44	15	919	3,215	804	2,411	911	260
3:00	6:52	50	18	1,060	3,179	795	2,384	884	295
2:30	5:44	60	21	1,257	3,142	785	2,356	856	343
2:10	4:35	69	24	1,439	3,117	779	2,338	838	387

An estimate of the calories needed to run a marathon at different speeds on a flat and windless course for a 70-kg (154-lb.) person. The total calories burned and estimate of calories from fat versus carbohydrate are calculated assuming that 75 percent of the calories burned are derived from carbohydrate. Based on an estimated 1,500 Calories of stored glycogen in active muscle (i.e., muscles used for running), the total carbohydrate that must be consumed is estimated by subtracting calories from glycogen.

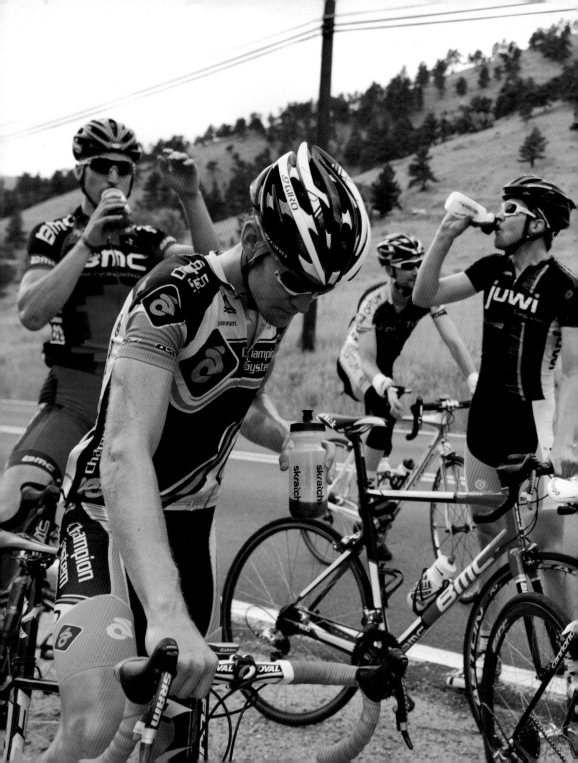

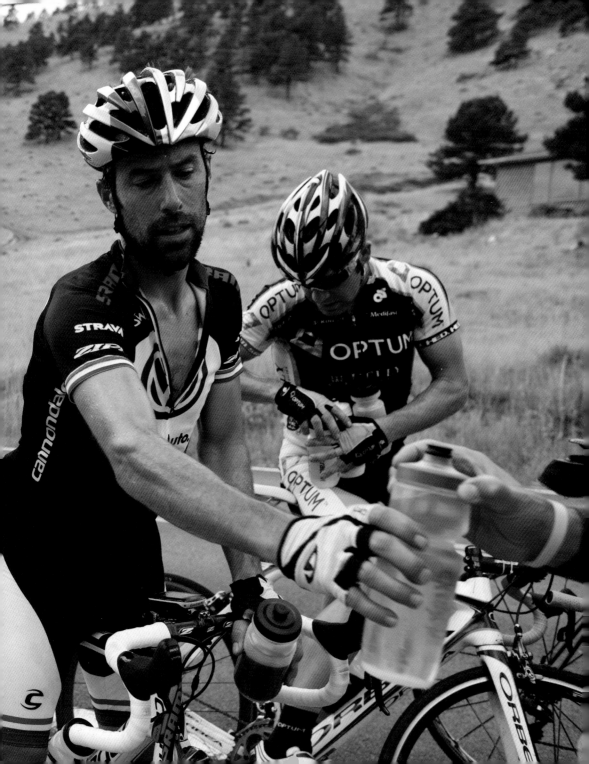

HYDRATION› WHY SWEAT MATTERS

While it's important to know how many calories we might need during exercise, when it comes to performance, fluid and electrolyte replacement is equally, if not more, important. In the same way that we can live without food for weeks and survive only days without water, performance depends more on hydration than it does on food.

Our performance can suffer with even a small amount of dehydration, even if we have plenty of energy on board to keep us going. At even a slight fluid loss equivalent to 2 percent of one's body weight, performance can begin to drop with noticeable declines in power and speed occurring at 3 to 4 percent of body weight loss. After a 5 percent body weight loss, there is a real risk for heat-related injuries as well as illness due to the dehydration itself. Gastrointestinal distress, lethargy, fatigue, confusion, shock, seizures, and even death can result from severe dehydration and increases in core temperature. Though it's a terrible thing to run out of fuel and bonk during exercise, bonking is seldom life-threatening, whereas dehydration can be. By the time someone reaches a 10 percent body weight loss due to dehydration, it is very likely he or she is facing a medical emergency.

Dehydration due to sweating results in both a loss of fluid and electrolytes. Sweat contains a number of different electrolytes including sodium, chloride, potassium, magnesium, and calcium. Sodium and chloride are the most depleted by far. Between these two electrolytes, sodium is the most critical with respect to how the body functions.

We can lose anywhere from 600 to 1,200 mg of sodium for every liter of sweat loss. If we only drink water, we dilute the sodium concentration in our blood, putting ourselves at risk for a low blood sodium level, something referred to as hyponatremia. Hyponatremia can cause a host of problems, ranging from fairly benign symptoms like fatigue, confusion, and headaches to severe issues like seizures, incontinence, and even death. Needless to say, it's important, if not vital, that when you exercise you drink fluids with a concentration of sodium that is similar to what you lose in sweat or that you pair your water with foods that contain a high salt content.

Since sodium loss in sweat is variable, it can be hard to know how much sodium to actually consume. Sometimes salt is visible on clothing or skin after a hard workout. While not an exact measurement, visual clues can indicate if you are on the high or low side of salt loss. Another clue is frequency of urination. If you are losing a lot of salt and just drinking water, then your kidneys will sense the diluted sodium levels and begin filtering excess water, causing you to urinate. What results is a body weight drop due to dehydration that is also paired with a paradoxical and consistent need to pee. If you are drinking a lot but still losing a significant amount of body weight because of dehydration and also find yourself needing to urinate a lot, then it's quite likely that you are not getting in enough sodium.

On average, the sweat rate of most endurance athletes in cool to moderately hot temperatures can range from 1 to 2 liters per hour and in very hot weather, as much as 4 liters per hour. If you think that calculating how many calories we need to eat during exercise is complicated, predicting how much a person sweats is a mathematical corn maze. There are environmental factors like temperature, humidity, solar radiation, and barometric pressure. There are also physiological and anatomical factors like one's metabolic rate, core temperature, skin temperature, body mass, and body surface area to consider. Finally,

EXERCISE HYDRATION MIX FROM SKRATCH LABS

A sports drink is intended to replace the fluid and electrolytes that are lost in sweat while also providing a quick hit of simple sugar to help fuel the working muscles. It can be really difficult to find a sports drink with enough sodium that isn't syrupy sweet or full of excess ingredients—factors contributing to gastrointestinal (GI) distress.

Frustrated by this problem, I started making my own sports drink from scratch. With a captive audience of athletes training for the Tour de France, I began experimenting, trying to use only what I knew the athletes needed and nothing else.

After a lot of trial and error, I learned that a combination of sucrose and glucose worked best for maximizing gastric emptying and intestinal absorption. Sucrose is a simple sugar made of glucose and fructose. As other researchers have found, because glucose and fructose each have their own

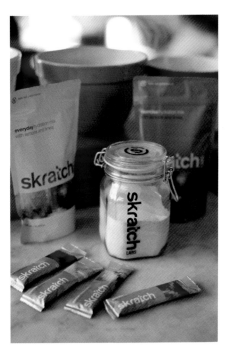

CONTINUED ON NEXT PAGE

there are a number of factors like heat acclimatization, clothing, and airflow that can have a huge impact on our sweat rate.

But unlike measuring our metabolic rate and energy expenditure, which requires expensive laboratory equipment and access, we can measure our fluid loss with something cheap and available to all of us—a scale. Though not perfectly exact because of the fuel we also burn during exercise, for the most part the weight we lose during exercise is water weight. You just need to know that 1 pound of water is equal to about 15.4 ounces of water and that 1 kilogram (2.2 lbs.) of water is equal to 1 liter of water.

By weighing yourself before and after you exercise in different conditions you can

---

EXERCISE HYDRATION MIX FROM SKRATCH LABS *(CONTINUED FROM PREVIOUS PAGE)*

transporter in the small intestine, using these two sugars together optimizes the transport of fuel into the body. I also learned that the drink was optimal at no more than a 4 percent carbohydrate concentration (4 grams per 100 ml or 80 Calories per half-liter), which agreed with existing literature on exercise hydration and gastric emptying rates.

Next, I settled on 300 mg of sodium per half-liter serving—almost triple the sodium found in most sports drinks. While this is on the low side of the sodium loss in sweat, I wanted to be conservative because many of the foods we were giving the riders during events were high in salt. Interestingly, when we tried giving riders this amount of sodium using regular table salt or sodium chloride in the solution, they complained it left a bad feeling in their mouths and stomachs. Using table salt with food didn't cause any problems. So we started using sodium citrate in the drink mix, which eliminated the problem. Citrate is essentially citric acid or lime juice with the acid removed, leaving a negative ion that pairs easily with sodium. It's easy on the stomach, is a strong acid buffer, and has a good taste, so we used citrate for all of our electrolytes, which also included potassium, calcium, and magnesium at concentrations similar to sweat.

Finally, I decided to let nature flavor the drink, and simply added some freeze-dried fruit powder. This eliminated the need for excess ingredients like food coloring, emulsifiers, flavoring agents, or fire retardant. The final product was a light-tasting exercise hydration mix that could be consumed at very high volumes without complaints of GI distress. At an osmolality of 160 mOsm per kg, the resulting drink is extremely hypotonic and in both theory and in practice empties and absorbs rapidly from the stomach and small intestine. After making batches by hand for years, I launched Skratch Labs with a group of friends to share our all-natural sports drink with athletes around the world. To learn more or purchase some for yourself, go to **www.skratchlabs.com**.

learn how well you are hydrating, and this feedback can give you a better sense of how much to drink for different effort levels and environments. Leading up to the 2008 Tour de France, I had riders weigh themselves constantly before and after their workouts. By the time they got to the Tour, they were so well calibrated that they could tell me how dehydrated they were within half a percent without even stepping on a scale.

To better understand the effect of hot temperatures and high-calorie drinks on hydration, let's take a look at how our bodies digest and process the calories we eat and drink.

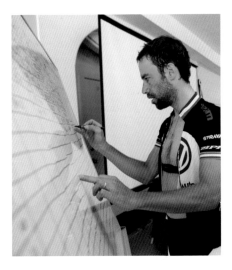

WHY NOT JUST DRINK COCONUT WATER?

Admittedly, I have joined the craze of all-natural, real food, organic, do-it-yourself drinks and foods. Many in this camp have adopted coconut water as an all-natural or real-food sports drink. While I understand the spirit of this decision, the rationale is ridiculous.

Why? Because coconut water does not come remotely close to having an electrolyte profile that is similar to sweat. We lose primarily sodium in sweat in amounts ranging from 600 mg to 1.5 grams per liter, and coconut water has almost no sodium in it. As for potassium, there is only 50 to 100 mg of potassium in a liter of sweat, and coconut water is chock full of it, with about 1,200 mg per liter. This is exactly the opposite of what you actually need to replace when you are dehydrated as a result of sweat loss.

The other problem with coconut water is that in large or sudden doses, potassium can actually be dangerous, leading to heart arrhythmias and other imbalances that can affect electrical signals across nerves as well as the chemical equilibrium of body cells. In fact, if you were to inject 3 grams of potassium into your body at once—the equivalent of 2.5 liters of coconut water—you'd probably end up dead. Luckily, it's pretty difficult and probably not appealing for most people to chug 2.5 liters of coconut water at one time.

Still, I know people who are obsessed with drinking coconut water as an all-natural sports drink. Just realize that coconut water isn't a sports drink and it's not something that I would ever advise as the sole means of replacing the fluid you lose from sweat.

THE MILLION-DOLLAR QUESTION›
DO WE DRINK OR EAT OUR CALORIES?

A lot of people come to the conclusion that since hydration is paramount, they should just drink their calories during prolonged endurance exercise. To hit their caloric target, many athletes use a high-calorie sports drink or semisolid gels, which often lead to complaints of gastrointestinal distress. If you've never had a problem with these products, consider yourself lucky and keep on doing what works for you. But if you've ever experienced gastrointestinal problems like bloating, stomach upset, vomiting, or diarrhea during exercise—a syndrome that many athletes refer to as "gut rot"—drinking or consuming solutions that are very high in calories may be a big part of the problem.

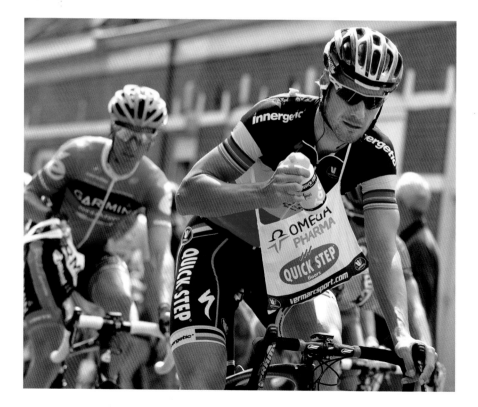

On the surface, it seems reasonable to assume that a calorie is a calorie regardless of form and that 200 Calories in a liquid state is the same as 200 Calories of a solid portable food. Moreover, it seems even more reasonable to assume that semisolid liquids and gels are preferred because they're already broken down and should be able to move faster through our stomach into the small intestine, where water and nutrients are ultimately absorbed. These high-calorie solutions, however, can be extremely difficult to tolerate because they can actually slow the transport of fluid, inhibit the movement of water across the small intestine, and directly irritate and overwhelm your gut, especially when you are dehydrated, stressed, or hot.

While I'd love for you to just take my word for it, to completely understand how a highly concentrated drink or gel can

A SLIGHT DETOUR INTO THE BOWELS

Although we often think of our muscles, heart, and lungs as the most important organs for athletic performance, our gastrointestinal tract, or GI tract for short, can make or break performance. Like all of our organ systems, the GI tract is put through a lot of stress when we're on the move and can be negatively affected by increases in body temperature, dehydration, and diversions in blood flow that occur during exercise. During exercise the process of digestion and absorption is not principally different than it is at rest. In fact, this process is robust enough to handle most exercise situations, but it can be compromised by prolonged exercise, especially in the heat, and if not managed properly, it can dismantle one's performance.

The GI tract is not technically the inside of our body—it's basically just a hol-

These high-calorie solutions can be extremely difficult to tolerate because they can actually slow the transport of fluid, inhibit the movement of water across the small intestine, and directly irritate and overwhelm your gut, especially when you are dehydrated, stressed, or hot.

wreak havoc on our body during exercise, let's diverge into the bowels for some basic gastrointestinal physiology. Once we have some background on how water and nutrients are actually digested and absorbed, we can explore the best ways we've discovered for getting enough fuel and hydration when exercising.

low tube going through us that is exposed on both ends to the outside world. Anatomically, the major components of this tube that play a role in processing what we consume are the mouth, stomach, small intestine, and large intestine. So as a point of clarification when we talk about nutrients or water being assimilated by the body, I'm referring to food or drink already in your gut being absorbed into circulation with blood through the very thin membrane that makes up your small intestine.

We often try to shove food past our mouth as quickly as possible when we are down carbohydrates, fats, and proteins. The net result is that a bolus entering the stomach is eventually turned into a liquid called *chyme*. That chyme is then trickled through the pyloric sphincter at the bottom of the stomach into the small intestine.

The emptying rate for a liquid is distinct from the emptying rate of a bolus, or chewed piece of food, even though liquid and solid foods can mutually affect gastric emptying rates because of the mixing action of the stomach.

exercising, but the mouth plays a key role in the first step of the digestive process by breaking apart food through chewing. That chewed food is called a bolus and is mixed with saliva, which lubricates the bolus and contains the enzyme amylase that helps to break down carbohydrates. The mouth also plays a key role in tasting our food and drink and making sure we aren't putting something foul into our belly. The process of chewing also sends signals to prep the stomach and small intestine for incoming food.

Once a bolus of food or any fluid is swallowed, it flows down our esophagus past our esophageal sphincter into our stomach. The stomach essentially serves as a large reservoir and has an undistended capacity of about 1 liter, though it can stretch when full to as much as 3 liters. Almost no absorption of water or nutrients occurs in the stomach. The main role of the stomach is to hold, mix, and digest food that enters it by releasing an array of enzymes and stomach acid that breaks

This process of mixing and digestion within the stomach can take as little as fifteen minutes or as long as a few hours, depending upon the type of food consumed. For example, a steak is going to take a lot longer to break down and digest than a cupcake. The length of time it takes for a bolus or liquid to pass through the stomach into the small intestine is referred to as the *gastric emptying rate* (GER). Because digested contents need to be emptied from the stomach before any absorption can take place, the gastric emptying rate is the first rate-limiting step in fueling and hydration. It's important to realize that the emptying rate for a liquid is distinct from the emptying rate of a bolus, or chewed piece of food, even though liquid and solid foods can mutually affect gastric emptying rates because of the mixing action of the stomach. For example, the gastric emptying rate of water is slowed by the presence of a chewed piece of steak but still greater than the steak itself. So if we drink a glass of water while eating a piece of food, much of that water will be out of the stomach before the food is.

Beyond the type of food eaten, gastric emptying is affected by a host of other variables including what we drink, the intensity of our effort, and our general state of being.

WHAT SLOWS DOWN GASTRIC EMPTYING RATE› High-intensity exercise (above 70–80% of max) ★ Increased body temperature ★ **Dehydration** ★ High psychological stress ★ **Reduced volume of liquid** ★ **High caloric density in food and drink** ★ Warm drink temperature ★ High fiber content ★ Low moisture content in foods

WHAT SPEEDS UP GASTRIC EMPTYING RATE› Lower exercise intensity ★ Regulating body temperature ★ **Hydration** ★ Low psychological stress ★ **Increased volume of liquid** ★ **Lower caloric density in food and drink** ★ Very cold drink temperature ★ Low fiber content ★ High moisture content in foods

Where food and drink are concerned, the main factors that slow gastric emptying are foods or liquids with a high-caloric density, higher fiber content, large particle size, and foods high in protein and fat. Gastric emptying is, in general, also slower in women than men. By increasing the volume of liquid entering the stomach, lowering the caloric density of your food and drink, and in some cases using a very cold drink temperature, you can speed up gas-

tric emptying. Ultimately, of all the factors that affect the gastric emptying rate, the three most important are all related to hydration. A low water volume entering the stomach, high caloric density, and a body that is dehydrated will all slow gastric emptying and hamper the speed at which water and nutrients can be absorbed by the body.

Everything emptied from the stomach enters the small intestine, which is the primary site for the actual absorption of water, nutrients, and electrolytes into the body. The small intestine also functions as the gut's main protective barrier, selectively transporting what we need while keeping harmful substances out of the body. Although the small intestine is contained in a very small space, when extended it is 16 to 32 feet in length with a surface area of 2,000 to 3,000 square feet—the size of a tennis court. This large surface area gives the small intestine an incredible capacity for absorption thanks to all of the folds within the small intestine and tiny hairlike structures called microvilli that extend from the individual cells, or enterocytes, that make up the intestinal wall. These cells are linked together by specialized proteins that form tight junctions to maintain the gut barrier; along with the intestinal cells, they help regulate the transport of substances.

Once the liquid chyme is inside the small intestine, the process of digestion continues as enzymes from the intestinal wall, pancreas, and liver are released into the lumen, or intestinal space, to further break down proteins, fats, and carbohydrates into their most basic elements. Proteins are broken down into individual amino acids or very small peptide chains, fats or triglycerides are broken down into free fatty acids and glycerol, and carbohydrates are broken down into individual sugar molecules like glucose or fructose.

The small intestine acts as a semipermeable membrane, allowing water to move freely across it, while actively regu-

Molar concentration is the number of individual molecules or solutes that are dissolved in water. This number is independent of the size or mass of the molecules and with respect to water movement is normally referred to as the *osmotic pressure* or osmolality of a solution measured in milliosmoles per kilogram of water (mOsm per kg). In effect, measuring the osmolality or osmotic pressure of a solution is like counting the number of people on a plane

A low water volume entering the stomach, high caloric density, and a body that is dehydrated will all slow gastric emptying and hamper the speed at which water and nutrients can be absorbed by the body.

lating the transport of certain molecules, nutrients, and electrolytes through specific gates or channels. Once foodstuffs are completely digested by the small intestine, they are primarily transported through an energy-dependent process called active transport, which moves substances "uphill" against a concentration gradient. This investment of energy ensures that nutrients get absorbed into the body rather than flow out of the body into the gut. In contrast, water moves passively across the small intestine in either direction through a process called osmosis. Put simply, osmosis is the movement of water across a semipermeable membrane from an area of low molar concentration to an area of high molar concentration. Water follows the crowd, flowing toward the side of the small intestine with the greatest number of stuff (molar concentration).

without concern for their size or weight. In the world of osmosis, 100 pregnant women on one side of the aisle have the same osmolality and attraction for water as 100 small children on the other side of the aisle as long as they each are completely dissolved in water or "buckled in." I'll use the terms *concentration, osmotic pressure,* and *osmolality* interchangeably to describe how much "stuff" is dissolved in a given solution and its effect on the movement of water.

Although the active transport of nutrients in the small intestine is separate from the passive movement of water, it's important to realize that the two are tightly linked. For the most part, it's the active transport of nutrients and electrolytes across the intestinal membrane that creates and maintains the osmotic gradient or concentration difference that pulls water into the body. As digested food-

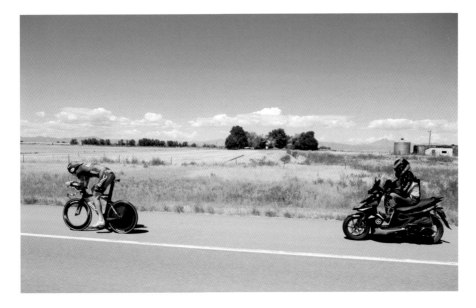

stuff gets transported into the body, the osmolality of fluid in the intestinal lumen decreases while the osmolality of blood in the body increases. Since water always flows toward the side with the highest concentration, the establishment of the concentration difference by the active transport of nutrients into the body causes water to follow suit and flow into the body. It's possible, however, for water to move in either direction. For example, if active transport systems were overwhelmed by a highly concentrated liquid, water would flow out of the body into the small intestine until those transport systems were able to restore the osmotic gradient.

Beyond osmosis, a small amount of water can also be co-transported or pulled into the body during the active transport of sodium and glucose. Specifically, the transport of 2 molecules of sodium and 1

molecule of glucose pulls 210 molecules of water in with it. This is why drinks with a little bit of sugar and a fair amount of sodium can increase the speed of water absorption compared to water alone. Still, in a 1,000-ml solution with 1 gram of sodium and 4 grams of glucose, this mechanism would pull in only about 100 ml, or 10 percent of the water. So osmosis is really the primary mechanism for moving water across our intestinal membrane, from the interior of our gut into our body.

After nutrients and water are transported into the body by the small intestine, anything that can't be digested or absorbed flows into the large intestine, where bacteria break down undigested material and where excess water is reabsorbed to form fecal matter. The rest is just nature taking its course—the grand departure—something we are all familiar with.

SHORTCUTTING THE BOWELS

If you skipped past the bowels, here are the highlights:

1 **The gastrointestinal system is the critical portal for fuel and hydration,** and for that reason it is one of the most important organ systems allowing us to sustain prolonged endurance exercise.

2 **Getting that food and water is a process that begins with chewed** food forming a bolus in our mouth, being swallowed, and moving into our stomach along with anything we drink. The stomach acts as a temporary reservoir where everything is mixed and digested to form a liquid called chyme.

3 **The length of time it takes food and liquid to pass through the stomach is termed the gastric emptying rate,** and it can vary based upon the type and amount of food, the caloric density of liquid, volume of liquid, and factors that affect our body like dehy-dration, body temperature, and exercise intensity.

4 **Once chyme enters the small intestine, it continues to be digested.** When nutrients are completely broken down, they are moved or absorbed across the small intestine using energy-dependent active transport systems. In contrast, water moves passively in either direction across the small intestine, freely moving toward the side with the highest concentration or osmotic pressure. This concentration, or osmotic gradient, is in part determined by the active transport of nutrients across the small intestine and by the osmolality of fluid entering the small intestine.

5 **Finally, any excess food or water that isn't absorbed moves down** the large intestine and eventually out the "back door."

BACK TO EATING AND DRINKING

So what's the best way to both fuel and hydrate? To answer that question, it's important to consider both gastric emptying and intestinal absorption, since both are critical pieces in the delivery of fuel and hydration. Fundamentally, to know whether you should eat or drink you need to determine if you are losing fluid faster through sweat than you are burning calories or if you are burning calories faster than you are sweating.

If we just look at gastric emptying and do not consider factors that affect intestinal absorption, it is clear that drinking more while keeping the carbohydrate concentration low is a key first step that will maximize our ability to both fuel and hydrate. In fact, if we are solely drinking water and not eating, the maximum gastric emptying rate of the stomach is about 2.5 liters per hour. This rate is maintained for low-ence a 3 percent deficit or more in body weight due to dehydration. These riders are able to empty and absorb up to 3 liters per hour, which exceeds what is normally thought of as the maximal gastric emptying rate. To keep up that rate, using a standard 600-ml (20-oz.) water bottle, these riders have learned that they liter-

Fundamentally, to know whether you should eat or drink you need to determine if you are losing fluid faster through sweat than you are burning calories or if you are burning calories faster than you are sweating.

calorie drinks up to a 4 percent carbohydrate solution (40 grams of carbohydrate per liter of water). So at our maximum rate of fluid intake, our maximum rate of carbohydrate delivery is about 100 grams per hour. When we increase the calories to have a 6 percent solution, gastric emptying drops to about 1.8 liters per hour. At this slightly higher concentration the volume of water that we can deliver is 28 percent lower, and in return the rate of carbohydrate entering into the small intestine is only 8 percent greater, at 108 grams per hour. Finally, with a high-caloric drink or 10 percent solution, maximal gastric emptying is reduced to about 1.5 liters per hour. This drops fluid delivery by 40 percent but boosts carbohydrate to 50 percent, or 150 grams per hour.

Hot days push the limits

For perspective on gastric emptying rates, I've personally observed riders on hot days in the Tour de France drink up to 25 bottles in a 5-hour stage and still experi-ally need to chug half to nearly a whole water bottle per gulp. With 96 Calories per bottle at a 4 percent solution, that's 2,400 Calories consumed through drink. If this were a hard day on the Tour, the average energy expenditure would be about 4,000 Calories. Knowing that a rider has at least 1,500–2,000 Calories of glycogen on board, most of the needed energy could, in this scenario, be replaced just with liquid calories. We often think of something like a rider's maximal oxygen consumption as rate-limiting performance in endurance events like the Tour, but on a hot day, it's really a well-adapted gut and the tireless work of domestiques retrieving water bottles that keeps the peloton moving.

Like riders in the Tour de France, many endurance runners can also experience sweat rates in excess of 3 liters per hour. Unfortunately, drinking a lot of fluid when running can be uncomfortable because of the physical pounding and the discomfort associated with water sloshing in the stom-

TABLE 6› LIQUID VS. SOLID CALORIES: It Depends on the Temperature

		COOL TEMPERATURES				HOT TEMPERATURES			
TIME hrs:min.	CARBS NEEDED TO EAT	Sweat Rate (L per hr.)	# Bottles	Liquid Calories	Solid Calories	Sweat Rate (L per hr.)	# Bottles	Liquid Calories	Solid Calories
6:30	761	0.8	4.6	446	315	1.5	10.5	1,004	0
6:00	1,058	0.9	5.7	549	509	1.8	12.6	1,210	0
5:30	1,439	1.2	7.1	681	759	2.3	15.4	1,474	0
5:10	1,758	1.4	8.2	791	967	2.7	17.6	1,694	64
4:50	2,144	1.6	9.6	925	1,219	3.3	20.4	1,961	183
4:30	2,619	2.0	11.3	1,089	1,530	4.0	23.9	2,290	329
4:10	3,090	2.4	13.0	1,252	1,838	4.8	27.2	2,616	475

Without changing your bike drafting position, this would be very difficult.

Sweat rate estimates for cool temperatures (50–70°F), where 25 percent of the heat lost is via sweat or evaporation, and for hot temperatures (70–90°F), where 50 percent of the heat lost is through evaporation of sweat. Based on these sweat rates and allowing for a 3 percent fluid weight loss, the number of 600-ml (20-oz.) bottles needed are calculated along with the calories coming in liquid form versus the number of calories that would be needed from solid food.

ach. There isn't a difference in the gastric emptying rate between activities, at least not in theory. However, we know that if a runner does not drink enough, the gastric emptying rate will inevitably slow due to the lower volume of fluid and the onset of dehydration. This sets up a vicious cycle of more dehydration and more impaired delivery. The net result is that most endurance runners are more likely to fall apart because of GI distress and dehydration than from a lack of fuel.

In thinking about a person's sweat rate versus his or her caloric needs, it's rare, as we discussed earlier (see Tables 4 and 5), to ever need more than 100 grams or 400 Calories of carbohydrate per hour. At the same time, it can be very easy to lose quite a bit of sweat during exercise depending upon the temperature. To put this into context, in Table 6, I expanded the esti-mates for calories required during a 100-mile bike ride, from Table 4, to also include estimates for sweat loss during cool (50 to 70°F) and hot temperatures (70 to 90°F). These sweat rates were calculated by esti-mating the amount of heat produced for the different power outputs and making some assumptions about the amount of cooling from evaporative sweat loss as well as other mechanisms such as wind flow. With the myriad variables at play it's not a perfect calculation, but the estimates are at least proportional to increases in work-load. Allowing for a 3 percent body weight loss, I then estimated the number of 600-ml bottles that would be needed as well as the calories that would be consumed using a 4 percent carbohydrate solution (4 grams of carbohydrate per 100 ml = 96 Calories per 600-ml bottle)—a concentration that would not impair gastric emptying. The net result is a breakdown of the maximum number of calories that you can get from a low-calorie drink and the remaining calories that would need to be delivered either with food or a higher calorie drink.

These estimates show that in cool temperatures, because of the lower sweat rates (1 to 1.5 liters per hour) only about half of the calories required can be provided from a low-calorie 4 percent carbohydrate solution. In theory the rest would need to come from either food or a higher carbohydrate solution. Knowing

more an issue of logistics than ignorance. We don't all enjoy the luxury of a support vehicle or faithful domestique. We may know what to do, but getting it done is a whole other issue that we as a community of race organizers, coaches, and athletes need to address. But that's a discussion for another time and place.

If we drink enough in hot situations to stay relatively hydrated using a 4 percent carbohydrate solution, we can meet our energy needs. But for those times when we need more calories than a low-

It's clear that in the heat most of us need to be drinking more, not eating more. If we were to keep up with our fluid loss, we could also keep up with our energy expenditure—even with a lower calorie drink.

that the maximal gastric emptying rate for a 10 percent solution is about 1.5 liters per hour, it's theoretically possible for the stomach to deliver enough water and calories through a higher calorie solution, but this depends on whether absorption in the small intestine can also keep pace.

In hot temperatures, if a person were to actually get access to enough sports drink to stay hydrated, even at a relatively low 4 percent concentration, in most situations, by just drinking there would be enough calories to meet the demand for energy. It's clear that in the heat most of us need to be drinking more, not eating more. If we were to keep up with our fluid loss, we could also keep up with our energy expenditure—even with a lower calorie drink. The only problem is that getting that much fluid is

concentration carbohydrate solution can provide or when we just can't access a lot of water, can we simply add more calories to the water we do have? As far as the stomach is concerned, the answer is probably yes, because the situations that call for more caloric density (which can hamper water delivery) are typically cooler situations when hydration is less critical. But the real question is whether the small intestine can adequately absorb a fuel cocktail with significantly less water.

Can absorption keep up with delivery?

Even though the active transport of nutrients or fuel eventually creates a concentration difference across the intestinal membrane that favors water movement into the body, water can sometimes move faster via osmosis across the small intestine than nutrients or electrolytes can be actively transported. This is especially the case when the gut is suddenly hit with a solution with a very high concentration or osmolality. When the osmolality of fluid reaching the small intestine is significantly greater than the osmolality of blood, the water inside the body will initially flow across the membrane into the gut, which can temporarily cause bloating and gastrointestinal distress. This means you're effectively dehydrating before rehydrating.

This backflow will continue until the small intestine is able to actively transport enough nutrients and electrolytes into the body to reverse the osmotic gradient across the membrane so that water is drawn back into the body. While the active transport of nutrients will eventually create an osmotic pressure that favors the movement of water back into the body, the temporary bloating or traffic jam initially caused by a highly concentrated solution can create a very uncomfortable feeling in the gut—a vicious cycle of back-and-forth traffic, which can also inhibit and slow the

FAILURE OF THE GUT BARRIER

The most common complaints I hear from endurance athletes revolve around gastro-intestinal distress, or "gut rot," during endurance events. At times, simply quitting seems to be the only remedy. This has led a number of physiologists to ask if the gut is actually well-equipped for prolonged endurance exercise and to wonder if the strength of one's intestinal membrane is a key rate-limiting factor in ultraendurance events.

Although the gut can handle most exercise situations, the intestinal barrier or gut barrier can fail during extreme and prolonged physical exertion. Factors that can increase the risk of this include a significant and prolonged decrease in blood flow and oxygen delivery to the intestines (i.e., intestinal ischemia), a significant rise in

body temperature (hyperthermia), and dehydration, especially when paired with local irritants such as a very concentrated glucose mixture, viruses, or nonsteroidal anti-inflammatories (NSAIDs). These situations can literally break apart the integrity of the intestinal membrane as the proteins forming the tight junctions between intestinal cells become inflamed and dysfunctional, causing real structural changes that increase the permeability of the small intestine—the gut becomes leaky.

A leaky gut can have dire consequences—bloating, nausea, vomiting, diarrhea, and intestinal bleeding. In addition, bacteria from our intestinal lumen can spill into our bodies, since the essential barrier function of the gut is compromised. This can

net movement of both water and nutrients into the body. In some cases, the osmolality of fluid reaching a person's small intestine may be so great and so sudden that an excessive amount of water pours across the intestinal membrane back into the gastrointestinal tract, causing a literal flood that flushes all of the nutrients and electrolytes down a path that leads back toward the light, also known as diarrhea (see Failure of the Gut Barrier, page 32).

To avoid this unpleasant reality, make sure that whatever is entering your small intestine has an osmolality that is hypotonic, or less than 260 mOsm per kg. This will allow water to move from the inside of the small intestine back into the body since the osmolality of blood is 260–290 mOsm per kg. You'd probably still be okay if the fluid entering your small intestine is isotonic, or the same as blood, since active transport mechanisms could more easily establish a favorable osmotic gradient for water movement into the body. However, if you are drinking fluids with an osmolality much greater than 290 mOsm per kg, making it hypertonic, make sure you have your diapers on because

result in low-grade endotoxemia as bacteria seeps into the blood, infecting the body and causing illness, sepsis, and shock.

The failure of the gut barrier can be dangerous, but some of the key factors that put us at risk are preventable—specifically, our exercise intensity, body temperature, and hydration status, all of which can individually put extreme stress on our gut and are interconnected. If exercise intensity is too high, blood is shunted away from the GI tract to working muscle, which can create areas of ischemia. Exercise intensity is also tightly linked to body temperature. And since hyperthermia itself can cause the tight junctions in the small intestine to fall apart, it's critical to temper how hot you get in part by pacing yourself, properly acclimatizing to the heat, and using cooling aids such as ice—pouring cold water over your body, drinking ice-cold fluids, and wearing protective clothing to stay cool in hot weather. Proper hydration can help us from overheating, but dehydration alone can cause the intestinal membrane to fail.

As simple as this sounds, pacing yourself, staying cool, and not becoming dehydrated are three of the most important things you can do to make sure your gut doesn't fall apart on you when you're exercising. And if you know you are sensitive to potential irritants such as highly concentrated carbohydrate solutions and NSAIDs like aspirin or ibuprofen, then make sure you stay away from them, especially on days when you'll be making big efforts.

you might be playing a game of intestinal Russian roulette.

For perspective, the majority of commercial sports drinks (like Gatorade) have about a 6 percent carbohydrate solution (240 Calories per liter) and an osmolality of anywhere from 270 to 320 mOsm per kg, depending upon the coloring agents, preservatives, emulsifiers, and flavor agents used. Excess ingredients can increase the osmotic pressure for no clear benefit. These sports drinks are still close to isotonic or somewhat hypertonic, but they leave little room for error when it comes to hydrating and fueling. In contrast, the Exercise Hydration Mix from Skratch Labs is a 4 percent carbohydrate solution (160 Calories per liter) with an osmolality of only 160 mOsm per kg, which makes it extremely hypotonic and which favors both maximal gastric emptying from the stomach and water absorption

What you need to know about high-calorie drinks

High-calorie carbohydrate drinks don't necessarily need to have a high osmolality. In fact, a huge number of high-calorie carbohydrate drinks and gels use a complex carbohydrate called maltodextrin to increase the caloric density while still keeping the osmolality low. Maltodextrin is a long chain of glucose molecules linked together to form one big molecule. The number of glucose subunits in a given maltodextrin molecule can range from 3 to 20. Accordingly, compared to one molecule of glucose, a single maltodextrin molecule can have 3 to 20 times the energy density. And since osmolality is determined by the total number of molecules in a solution and not their size, shape, or energy density, a single molecule of maltodextrin that has 20 times

This high caloric value and low osmotic pull is perhaps one of the reasons why maltodextrin is one of the most ubiquitous ingredients in the world of pre-packaged sports nutrition.

at the small intestine (see Exercise Hydration Mix from Skratch Labs, page 19). On the other extreme, sugary sodas like Coke normally contain a 10 percent carbohydrate solution (400 Calories per liter) and have an osmolality greater than 700 mOsm per kg. While it's common practice for many athletes to drink Coke late in a race, unless they're also drinking water with it, they're probably asking for trouble.

the energy as a single molecule of glucose exerts the same osmotic pressure or pull on water as that single glucose molecule. This high caloric value and low osmotic pull is perhaps one of the reasons why maltodextrin is one of the most ubiquitous ingredients in the world of pre-packaged sports nutrition.

The only problem is that it's highly unlikely that the osmolality of a malto-

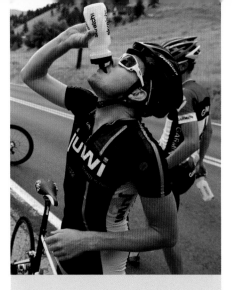

dextrin solution before it's consumed is the same once it's digested and sitting in the small intestine. Although many athletes are told and believe that using maltodextrin is a convenient way to drink more calories without upsetting their gut, by the time maltodextrin enters the small intestine and the process of digestion is nearly completed, most of that maltodextrin breaks apart into individual glucose units. In effect, what was once one molecule exerting only one molar equivalent of osmotic force breaks apart like a Trojan horse by the time the small intestine tries to absorb it. Theoretically, a maltodextrin drink with an osmolarity of 300 mOsm per liter before it's consumed could have an osmolarity as high as 6,000 mOsm per liter after it's digested. To understand what that would feel like in your gut, imagine a completely full flight with 300 pregnant women and mid-flight each of them giving birth to 20 screaming babies. That's a lot of little soldiers storming the intestinal wall. More realistically, 400 Calories in a 500-ml bottle (20 percent solution) using a maltodextrin made with a 20-unit glucose chain has a calculated osmolarity of 60 mOsm per liter of water. But, by the time it breaks down into individual glucose units at the level of the small intestine, the calculated osmolarity would be 1,110 mOsm per liter of water. Kind of makes those sugary sodas a lot more appealing.

DRINKING YOUR CALORIES

You can drink a fair amount of calories, but only up to a point. In **cooler weather,** when hydration is not a huge concern, **200 to 280 Calories per liter** of water (5–7% carbohydrate concentration) would probably work for most people. In **hot weather,** when hydration is a big concern, err on the low side of **140 to 180 Calories per liter** (3.5–4.5% carbohydrate concentration).

When evaluating different drink products, the easiest thing to do is keep the big picture in mind:

☆ **Look at the total calories**
☆ **Total amount of water per serving**
☆ **Total number of ingredients listed**

The higher the water content, the lower the calories, and the fewer the ingredients, the lower the osmotic pressure will be by the time that product is actually digested and reaches the small intestine for absorption into the body.

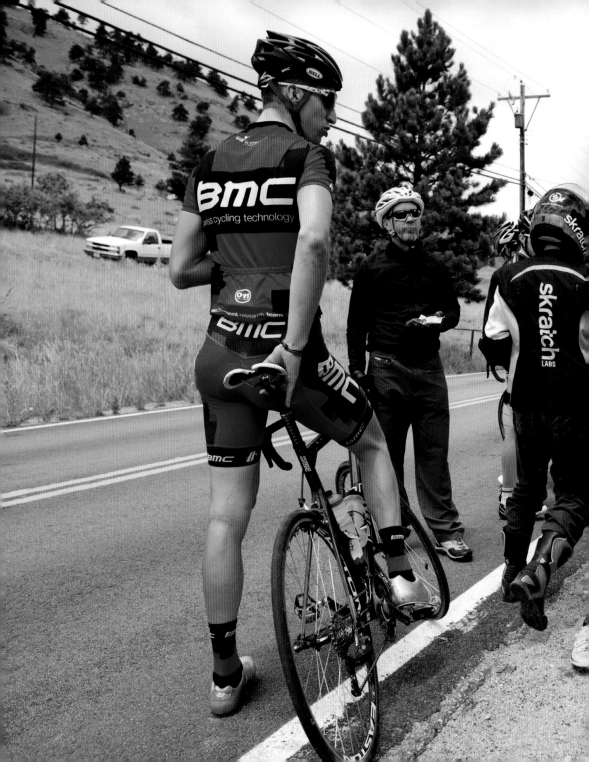

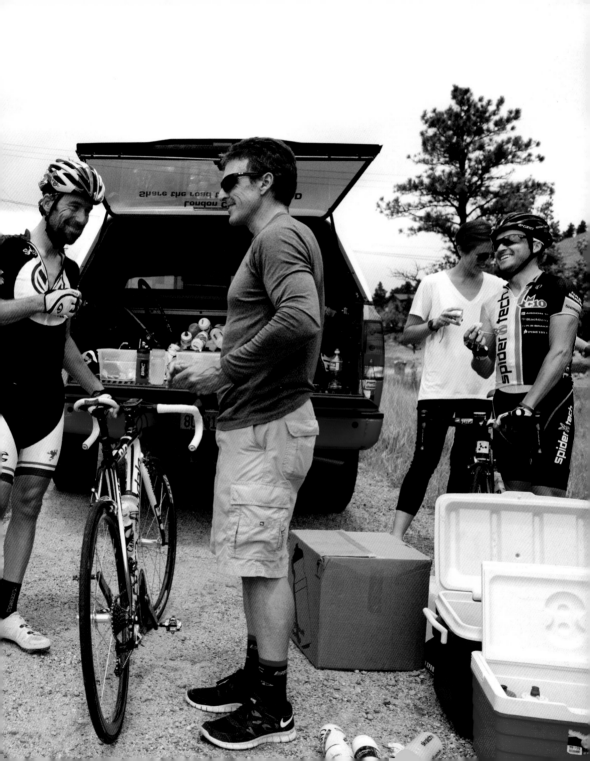

WHY SOLID FOOD IS NOT THE SAME AS LIQUID FOOD

While it's clear that the volume of high-calorie liquids we can safely ingest without the risk for gastrointestinal distress is limited as a result of their high osmolality, one major question remains—if we can't simply drink more calories, can we eat solid food to get those calories? We have only briefly touched on the idea that solid calories are different than liquid calories, but we have yet to figure out which is better. Wouldn't food digested in our body exert the same osmotic pressure once it's in the small intestine as a liquid product containing the same number of calories? Why not pour milk over our dinner and mix it all up—after all, it's going down the same pipe anyway.

First and foremost, solid food is fundamentally different from liquid food. As we discovered in the bowels, the main difference is that solid food has a slower gastric emptying rate compared to liquid food. Any food that is eaten must be digested and liquefied before it empties from the stomach, so if something starts out as a relatively solid albeit chewed mass, it will take longer for that food to digest and empty compared to the same amount of calories entering the stomach already in liquid form.

This might make it seem like eating food is a time-consuming way to get extra calories, and at first glance, this is true. Depending upon the food, it does generally take more time to get calories from solid

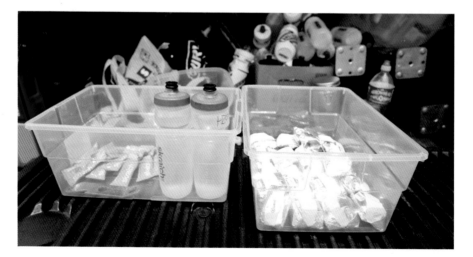

food into our bodies. Ironically, this is also why eating food can be a major advantage. Because food doesn't rapidly empty from the stomach, it also doesn't overwhelm the small intestine with a high volume of very concentrated chyme like high-calorie liquids or gels can, which can cause many ways, solid food is like a time-released energy capsule whereas high-calorie liquids are like instant-release energy gut-bombs.

Another advantage of keeping a reserve of calories from solid foods trickling in from the stomach is that it's less likely that our ability to hydrate will be impaired.

Another advantage of keeping a reserve of calories from solid foods trickling in from the stomach is that it's less likely that our ability to hydrate will be impaired.

water to flow into the gut via osmosis and cause bloating or GI distress. Solid food's slower emptying rate gives active transport mechanisms in the small intestine a chance to keep up with the transport of nutrients, and it allows the gut to maintain a favorable osmotic gradient to pull water back into the body. Drinking high-calorie liquids or gels is like unleashing a large number of cars onto the highway all at once, which can cause a traffic jam or accident. By contrast, eating solid food is like having a traffic light to regulate the flow of cars or calories onto a highway in a slower, more evenly paced fashion.

Continuing with this car analogy, one of the primary functions of the stomach is to act as a temporary parking lot or reservoir for food. By eating solid food, the stomach is able to reserve a store of calories that can be used over the course of an activity. Although these calories may not leave the stomach as quickly, they allow the stomach to act as an important caloric buffer. In

Though it is true that solid foods will slow the emptying of liquids and, conversely, liquids will speed the emptying of solid foods, because the digestion of food is not instantaneous, neither is the mixing of food and liquid. This means that if you take a bite of solid food and then also drink water with it, the water will empty faster through the stomach than the piece of food. Because food and drink can be disconnected at the level of the stomach, eating a piece of solid food doesn't immediately interfere or impair the movement of water, and this is a good thing. In stark contrast, if that same amount of energy was in liquid form, there wouldn't be a different emptying rate for either water or fuel. And as we discussed earlier, if that combination of water and fuel had a significantly greater osmolality than blood, we could be in trouble.

Athletes seem to have bought into the notion that during exercise they need energy sources that pass through the stomach as quickly as possible—that it would be easier on our GI tracts if we took the stress of digestion out of the picture. This notion is valid for short-duration high-intensity exercise. Having an empty stomach and relying on stored glycogen and even stored water may be optimal for short, hard performances. But during prolonged exercise it's advantageous to maintain a constant stream of energy Ironman triathlon—an event that can last well over eight hours—are conditioned to believe that avoiding solid food eases the pressure on our gut and that pre-packaged products that we wouldn't otherwise normally eat or enjoy are the right choice. If you have a hard time seeing yourself using these solutions and products while you're unstressed sitting around, but you don't

What does absolutely matter is that we manage how many total calories we consume and make sure we've got plenty of water and sodium to wash it all down.

rather than dealing with periodic influxes of energy. This is where the stomach, solid food, and normal digestion play a critical role. In fact, one of the advantages of being able to eat a solid meal a few hours before an endurance event is that we essentially top off our stomach, creating an additional energy reserve that can help steady the release of energy as we begin to exercise. Ultimately, the stomach is well adapted to handle food and water, to digest and serve as a reservoir. Trying to shortcut this simple function may create more problems than it solves.

Imagine what would happen if we consumed these high-calorie carbohydrate solutions and gels to meet the energy demands of an ordinary day instead of eating solid food. It's my guess that a lot of people wouldn't feel very good after eight hours of sucking down gels. Athletes competing in ultra-endurance events like an

hesitate to use them when you are stressed in the midst of an ultra-endurance event, it's time to rethink your approach. Either the rationale that these products are not stressful for the gut or the rationale that we need to bypass digestion is flawed. If something offends your belly when you are just sitting on the couch, don't expect that insult to magically go away when you are hiking, running, swimming, or riding.

With all of this distinction between solid versus liquid food in mind, there's one last idea I'd like to raise: despite everything I've just written, it's possible that it really doesn't matter one way or another what form our calories are in, so long as we stay hydrated and keep the net ratio or concentration of calories to water below a certain level. I've observed this phenomenon in a lot of endurance athletes—that on their best days they could literally eat whatever they wanted so long as they also drank a lot.

Curious about this, I asked Craig Alexander, three-time winner of the Ironman World Championships, what he consumed on his best race days. When he listed to me all of the gels, sodas, energy drinks, salt tablets, and blocks he normally consumes, I was shocked that his gut didn't completely unravel. But when we accounted for all of the water he drank on his good days and did some quick back-of-the-napkin math, we realized that if we took all of the calories he consumed, regardless of form, and all of the water he drank, his carbohydrate consumption was roughly 50 grams, or 200 Calories per liter of water—a 5 percent concentration. This is really close to the ideal mixture of water and fuel. On his bad days, however, what was very clear was that while Craig consumed the same number of calories, he did not drink nearly enough water.

Ultimately, the type of calories we use, whether solid or liquid, may all come down to personal preference—to what works for you. In the same way we can debunk the use of highly concentrated gels and liquids but concede that convenience sometimes takes precedence, we can also debunk the idea that we need to stay away from solid food during exercise and accept that eating what we enjoy can work just as well, if not better.

Despite all of the analysis, it's important to recognize that if all calories are equal, then there's a lot more to eating what we like—to eating what actually satisfies us than what is immediately apparent or that

I even understand or can quantify. Beyond the satiation we feel when our stomachs are full, there is a basic morale boost and sense of nourishment that good food can bring to us. When all is said and done, since everything we put down our throat does literally end up at the same place, it really may not matter if we pour milk all over our dinner and mix it up before we shove it down. But, what does absolutely matter is that we manage how many total calories we consume and make sure we've got plenty of water and sodium to wash it all down. For that reason, my personal preference, professional observation, and plain common sense tell me that managing the intake of food and drink using recipes, real foods, and products that taste good and that instinctively feel right works a lot better than trying to manage it with engineered nutrition pretending to be smarter than nature.

PRE-PACKAGED BARS VS. PORTABLES MADE FROM SCRATCH

Science can give us a clear rationale for eating solid food instead of relying on highly concentrated gels, semisolids, or liquids for calories. In practice, however, I've personally always had a hard time with many pre-packaged sports bars, and many athletes complain that they taste bad and hurt performance. This is what led me to make my own energy bars from scratch. I didn't really have the time or desire, but the homemade bars worked so much better. I was never quite sure why—I assumed that it was simply because the homemade stuff

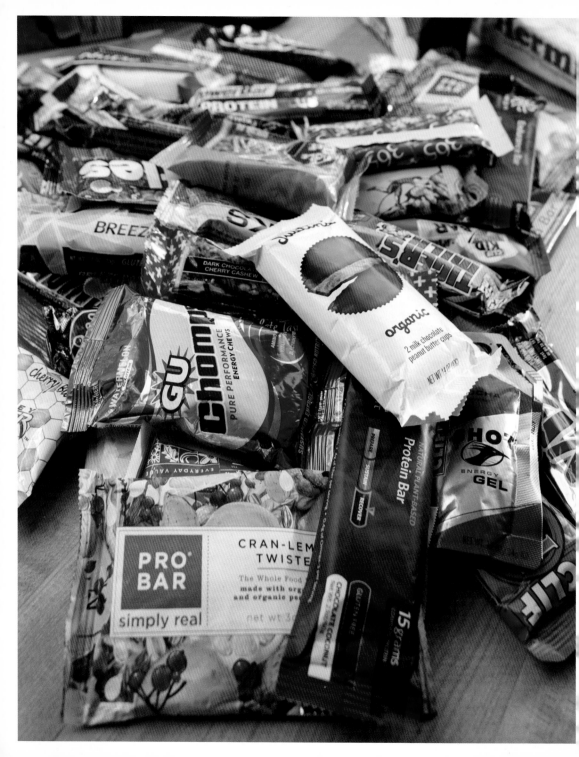

tasted better and had an intangible quality that came from being fresh, simple, and prepared with a lot of care.

While those intangible qualities may all be true and while that may be all there is to it, I wanted to find a stronger explanation for why rice cakes, little sandwiches, and waffles were better than what we could buy premade at the grocery store. With that goal in mind, I headed out to buy every pre-packaged bar, snack, or candy bar that could be potentially used as a portable food. By the time I got home, I had 11 different sports bars, 13 different candy bars, 6 fruit and nut bars, 6 protein bars, 3 cereal bars, 4 different types of "blocks," 5 different cookies, a rice crispy treat, 1 unfrosted cupcake, and 1 small bag of potato chips.

I compiled the nutrition facts—mass, total calories, carbohydrates, fat, protein, fiber, sodium, and the water content. I also decided to do something fairly unscientific and unobjective: I counted the total number of ingredients in each pre-packaged food item and then tallied the number of those ingredients that I recognized as an actual food. For example, if an ingredient was coconut, I counted it as "real." But for an ingredient such as polyglycerol polyriconoleate, I wouldn't count it because at a glance I had no idea what it was or where it came from. There was some gray area here. If an ingredient was something like soy protein isolate, I could deduce that it was probably just a processed soybean, but if I had to spend a lot of time thinking

about it, I was apt to deem it a nonfood. Finally, I divided the number of ingredients I recognized as real food by the number of total ingredients to get an impromptu metric based on my own ignorance that I called "percent real" (% Real).

I wanted to compare the nutritional breakdown of these pre-packaged products to the recipes in this cookbook. Because our recipes are made with real ingredients, the first distinction was easy—our portables are 100 percent real.

Table 7 lists the results of the analysis for each type of pre-packaged product, and Table 8 lists the results for each type of food included in this cookbook. As the data in the tables show, some of the major distinctions are revealed when we compare the average nutrition facts for the rice cakes in this cookbook against the sports bars I picked up at the grocery store.

PRE-PACKAGED FOOD VS. PORTABLES: HOW THEY STACK UP

	SPORTS BAR	RICE CAKES
Mass	54.5 g	138.1 g
Total calories	223	199
Carbohydrates	32.5 g	37 g
Fat (% cal.)	8 g (32%)	3.2 g (13%)
Protein	6.5 g	5.1 g
Fiber	3.5 g	1.3 g
Sodium	108 mg	101 mg
Water (% mass)	3.9 g (7%)	91.1 g (66%)

Note› Nutrition facts listed are an average of 11 leading sports bars and the 9 rice cake recipes featured in this book.

The difference in caloric content between the average sports bar and a rice cake is primarily due to the higher fat content of sports bars.

With respect to total calories, the average caloric content of a sports bar is slightly higher than a rice cake. The average sports bar, however, has significantly less carbohydrate and more fat. This reveals that the difference in caloric content between the average sports bar and a rice cake is primarily due to the higher fat content of sports bars (1 gram of fat adds up to 9 calories whereas 1 gram of carbohydrate is 4 calories). This difference is also due, in small part, to the slightly greater protein content found in the sports bars. Sodium values were nearly

the same. Looking at all of the sports bars, I counted an average of 18 different ingredients per bar and only recognized an average of 78 percent of them as real foods. In contrast, our rice cakes average 6 ingredients, all real.

All things considered, a sports bar isn't too different from a rice cake, until it comes to water content. Compared to the average sports bar, rice cakes have almost 23 times the total water content by mass (3.9 grams vs. 91.1 grams). To put this into perspective, if we think about these foods like we think about drinks (where

TABLE 7› Nutrition Facts for Pre-packaged Foods

TYPE (# in Sample)	INGREDIENTS Total #	INGREDIENTS % Real	MASS G wt.	TOTAL CAL.	CARB G	FAT G	FAT % Cal.	PRO G	FIBER G	Na+ MG	WATER G	WATER % Mass
Unfrosted Cupcake (1)	8.0	100%	100.0	264	42.0	9.0	31%	4.0	1.0	120	43.9	44%
Gel (5)	11.2	38%	37.8	106	24.4	0.6	6%	0.0	0.6	92	12.1	31%
Cookies (5)	16.0	76%	73.6	246	41.2	8.1	30%	3.0	0.9	87	20.3	22%
Block (4)	13.5	53%	49.5	160	39.5	0.0	0%	0.3	0.3	70	9.4	18%
Cereal Bar (3)	29.7	74%	41.3	160	29.7	3.7	21%	2.3	1.2	87	4.4	11%
Protein Bar (6)	19.3	59%	59.7	238	27.0	8.0	32%	17.0	2.2	170	5.3	9%
Soft Candy (2)	17.5	26%	60.1	240	51.5	3.8	14%	0.0	0.0	0	4.9	8%
Sports Bars (11)	18.1	78%	54.5	223	32.5	8.0	32%	6.5	3.5	108	3.9	7%
Potato Chips (1)	10.0	80%	56.8	280	36.0	14.0	46%	2.0	1.0	520	3.3	6%
Fruit & Nut Bar (6)	15.2	84%	50.7	223	26.0	12.0	47%	6.0	4.2	83	2.4	5%
Candy Bar (13)	17.5	50%	48.8	233	28.5	12.2	48%	4.2	1.5	102	2.1	4%

Compare to rice cakes in Table 8.

Nutrition breakdown of a variety of commonly found pre-packaged portable snacks and sports nutritionals. Each nutrition value is an average for that category.

100 grams of carbohydrate in 100 ml of water equals a 100 percent carbohydrate solution), we can assign a carbohydrate concentration to them in the same way that we assign that value to a drink like Coke (10 percent or 10 grams per 100 ml). Using this idea, the rice cakes would have a carbohydrate concentration of 40.6 percent while the sports bars would be an astounding 833 percent. This dense concentration, however, doesn't just apply to solid foods like sports bars. It also applies to semisolids like gels. For example, the average gel contains 24 grams of carbohydrate but only 12 grams of water (equivalent to 12 ml of water) but has a carbohydrate concentration of 203 percent.

Try our Sticky Bites, page 220.

THE DIFFERENCE WATER MAKES

Density and dryness explain why a lot of sports bars and gels are very hard to eat,

digest, and absorb, almost always requiring additional water. To understand how dry most sports bars are, imagine we are making a cake and after adding all of the dry ingredients into a bowl, we use only 10 percent of the water that the recipe requires before baking. What we would have at the end of the process would resemble a brick (or the typical sports bar), not a cake that we would want to serve for dessert or be excited to eat during a long endurance event. It's reminiscent of a time when sailors traveled by the power of wind and survived by eating hardtack—an extremely dry biscuit that was incredibly resistant to spoilage because it was made with flour, salt, and just a little bit of water. Hardtack was so hard and dry that sailors took to calling it tooth dullers, sheet iron, molar breakers, and dog biscuits—nicknames that

TABLE 8› **Nutrition Facts for Feed Zone Portables**

Compare to sports bars in Table 7

TYPE (# in Sample)	INGREDIENTS		MASS G wt.	TOTAL CAL.	CARB G	FAT		PRO G	FIBER G	Na+ MG	WATER	
	Total #	% Real				G	% Cal.				G	% Mass
Rice Cakes (9)	6.4	100%	138.1	199	37.0	3.2	13%	5.1	1.3	101	91.1	66%
Baked Eggs (6)	4.8	100%	97.0	127	6.7	6.7	49%	10.0	0.5	265	72.4	62%
Two-Bite Pies (8)	10.4	100%	82.0	184	24.2	7.6	35%	4.7	1.6	271	39.7	39%
Baked Cakes & Cookies (11)	7.9	100%	67.8	101	15.0	3.2	28%	3.2	0.7	225	44.2	46%
Griddle Cakes & Waffles (9)	6.4	100%	117.8	188	28.7	5.7	27%	5.6	1.6	210	64.5	45%
Aha! Portables (22)	6.8	100%	119.5	174	34.1	2.0	14%	4.0	1.2	126	78.1	54%
Take & Make (8)	6.8	100%	102.1	236	38.4	7.1	26%	5.9	2.0	208	46.7	42%

Nutrition breakdown for each major category of portable recipes included in this cookbook. Each nutrition value is an average for that category.

Reading a nutrition label isn't just about identifying the calories, carbohydrates, fats, and proteins anymore; it's a minefield that we creep across hoping that we don't step on an ingredient that explodes in our gut or that, even worse, prematurely kills us.

might be just as appropriate for a lot of the sports bars sold today.

Across the board, when I compare any of the pre-packaged foods I collected to a freshly made recipe, the single common difference is the water content. This is likely due to the need to increase the shelf life of pre-packaged foods. Without resorting to chemical preservatives, the easiest way to get a food to last unrefrigerated for a long time is to dry it out. It's an age-old technique used to preserve everything from meats to grains.

In a lot of ways, finding the balance between what to eat and drink is a puzzle right out of "Goldilocks and the Three Bears." Too many calories in liquid form and water doesn't empty from your gut. Too many calories in a dry solid form and the only thing that moves are venting gases. But just the right amount of calories and water in a delicious form and a balance is struck. It's a balance that has taken many athletes, including myself, a lot of time and tinkering to figure out through basic trial and error. A lot of that wasted time was a

DEHYDRATING TO REHYDRATE: A VOLATILE GAME

Dehydration is also a technique I once considered to make life easier while living on the road. Several years ago, I was brainstorming with Jonathan Coln, a former soigneur with the Garmin pro cycling team, about how to offer a greater variety of meals for the riders immediately after they got back onto the bus after a day of racing. It was extremely difficult if not impossible to cook on the bus, and I wanted to give the riders more than just a crusty old baguette sandwich and a protein drink after an event. So Jonathan suggested that we try dehydrated backpacking food. There was a local company that made a wide variety of meals for backpackers, and by just adding boiling water we could quickly serve something appealing like beef stroganoff, chicken and rice, or mashed potatoes and gravy. Studying the nutrition labels, we would at least be doing better than what the riders were currently eating, so Jonathan and I decided to pay the company a visit. We were suitably impressed after the tour of the facility and left with a handful of products to try. But as we were leaving, we were given a stern warning to make sure to rehydrate the food and not to get impatient or we might upset those around us. Not knowing what they were talking about, we went on our merry way.

consequence of an entrenched hubris that science, technology, and what is marketed to us are always better. As much as there needs to be a balance between the water and calories we consume, there needs to be a balance between what we consider to be new-school technocentric techniques and old-school ethnocentric views. It's a balance that says sometimes it's okay to try the middle bed despite the noisy claims made by the extremes on either side.

Extreme ingredients

Nowhere is one side of this extreme more apparent or scarier than when reading the ingredient list on most pre-packaged foods. While most ingredients are recognizable—flour, sugar, rice, oats, cocoa butter—so many, like brominated vegetable oil, carnauba wax, and carrageenan, are not recognizable without a chemical engineering degree or the patience to scour the Internet. In the limited time I spent researching some of these mystery ingredients, I became alarmed. I learned that tertiary butylhydroquinone, often listed as TBHQ, is a common food preservative but also an anticorrosive agent used in biodiesel that can cause stomach tumors and damage DNA in high doses. I found that malitol is a sugar alcohol typically used as a sugar substitute and, like many artificial sweeteners, can exert a laxative effect. Finally, I learned that xantham gum is used as a thickening

We returned to Jonathan's house excited to try our new meals. Good and hungry, we let the packages brew until our ignorance deemed ready and then chowed. Our initial response was that this wasn't bad; in fact, it might be a real possibility. But, within 30 minutes of polishing off our dinners, our bellies began erupting. What followed was the most intense and prolonged bout of flatulence either Jonathan or I have ever experienced in our adult lives. It was as if our gastrointestinal tracts had been converted into methane factories, tasked with creating energy for sentient machines that survived by turning pacified humans plugged into the Matrix into portable batteries. It was unreal, startling, and at times the pure comic majesty of the whole experience had me reveling in profound amazement and awe. Needless to say, we did not go through with this idea or ever mention it to anyone. We later learned that when food is not properly rehydrated before eating, as it rehydrates in the gut, it releases gases that can build pressure, cause bloating, and create volumes of free potential energy that would have made us wealthy if we could only have captured it. It's hard for me to not think about this experience every time somebody mentions that sports bars turn their stomach, driving others away from them.

agent and is made from the coating of the bacteria *Xanthomonas campestris*, which is responsible for causing black rot to form on leafy vegetables and broccoli. Overwhelmed, I gave up researching the rest of my list realizing that I could write an entire book on the ingredients used in prepackaged foods. And I had barely chipped the tip of the iceberg. When all of the chemical colors, flavoring agents, and even "natural" flavors are added to the mix, it becomes really hard to know what we are consuming or what the effects are on the body. Reading a nutrition label isn't just about identifying the calories, carbohydrates, fats, and proteins anymore; it's a minefield we creep across while hoping we don't step on an ingredient that will explode in our gut or, even worse, prematurely kill us.

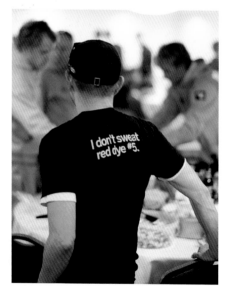

Real ingredients

The prevalence of unidentifiable ingredients is why I've become so fervent about cooking from scratch—about having control over the most basic ingredients we put into our body. This alone is reason enough to take the time to make your own foods to take with you when you're on the go rather than rely on prepackaged foods. There is a deep irony here—that eating foods that make our healthy lifestyle more convenient and easier may actually be making us sick. Likewise, when one takes a closer look at recipes like unfrosted cupcakes and cookies that are supposed to be bad for us, when we make them at home with real food ingredients, they may actually be much healthier for us compared to the processed equivalent, particularly when we're exercising and attempting to optimize our performance.

When all is said and done, I've learned that whether cooking at home or buying a ready-to-eat or -drink product from the store, simple is better. Choose products and recipes with a minimal number of ingredients, preferably real food, that you can recognize and that don't insult or challenge your intelligence even if they challenge your desire for convenience and insult a massive industry selling us quantity over quality. While I realize that this is a big "ask," life is full of compromises. We may not always be able to give ourselves the absolute best, but we deserve, at the very least, to do our best to try.

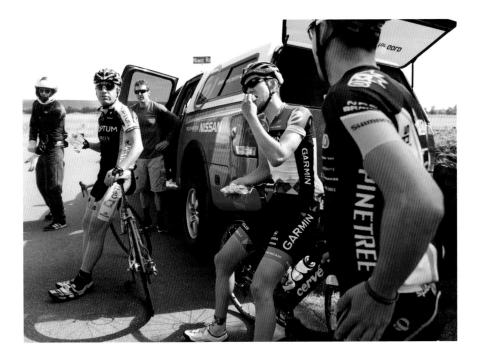

IT'S TIME TO JUST TRY

This book is an acknowledgment that we can't outsmart nature. It's an effort to keep things simple, share ideas, and further a discussion that we know has improved the health and performance of the athletes and friends we have cooked for. While I've learned through real-world experience that freshly prepared meals taste better and work better than pre-packaged alternatives, I'm hopeful that some of my analysis and rationale can convince more people to take action and try. Ultimately, this book is not about analysis, it's about finding the recipes and the time in our busy lives to slow down and enjoy the process of cooking food—to actually enjoy eating that food even if it's portable and

meant to be used while on the go to fuel our active lifestyles.

As much as I often attempt to reduce our nutrition to math and science, there is a larger aspect of science exhibited in food called emergence—the idea that the whole is much greater than the sum of its parts. It's a principle that has made me realize that it's not about robotically quantifying our nutritional needs. It's about remembering that we also eat and drink to nourish ourselves. And nourishment is something much greater than calories or individual ingredients. It's the soul in a great dish, pursuing a goal with close friends and family, and taking care of our entire being. Ask yourself if you're happy, if you're excited about the food that you're eating, and check in with yourself to see how you're feeling and how you're performing on a particular diet.

With this in mind, these recipes are a starting point for you to be your own scientific experiment. Despite all that a specific study can tell us, it is not the results but the scientific process that is what really matters. It's a process that we can all participate in to discover our own personal response. In every study there is always a range of outcomes—some positive, some negative, and many that are in the middle. Goldilocks had it right when she tried all three beds and found the one that was just right. In the end, you alone are responsible for your choices, and this book is a reminder to keep an open mind in the discovery process and to also stay committed to what you know works best for you.

That responsibility and discipline extends to putting our activity and our diets

Sugar and salt can kill us when eaten in excess as part of a sedentary lifestyle, but they can be amazing ergogenic aids and even lifesavers when we are in the middle of an extreme endurance event. It's all about context and the discipline and perspective it takes to keep things in context.

For this reason, we worked hard to create an extremely diverse list of recipes that range in their nutritional profile and that we think taste great. Some are higher in fat while others are not. Some are all about maximizing carbohydrate content while others are about extra protein. Similarly, we put each recipe to the test to make sure that our directions create what's pictured and described nutritionally. But, as Chef Biju often reminds me, no recipe is ever supposed to be religiously followed. Use them as a rough guideline or as inspiration to make something even better. Feel free to experiment—season

Nourishment is something much greater than calories or individual ingredients. It's the soul in a great dish, pursuing a goal with close friends and family, and taking care of our entire being.

into context. It's realizing that without proper training and consistent physical activity, no diet or nutrition plan will ever allow us to be our best. Likewise, a book of recipes, especially these recipes, won't do much for us unless we also remember to stay active. This is especially true since everything that might be good for us when we are exercising and sweating is likely bad for us when we are sitting on our butts.

and salt to your taste. Add less sugar or more according to what you like and feel you need. Be creative, and don't be discouraged if something doesn't quite work out as planned. For both Biju and me, the recipes and ideas here and in *The Feed Zone Cookbook* are a collection of successes born from countless unseen failures. Don't ever be afraid to fail, and may every recipe in this book bring you success.

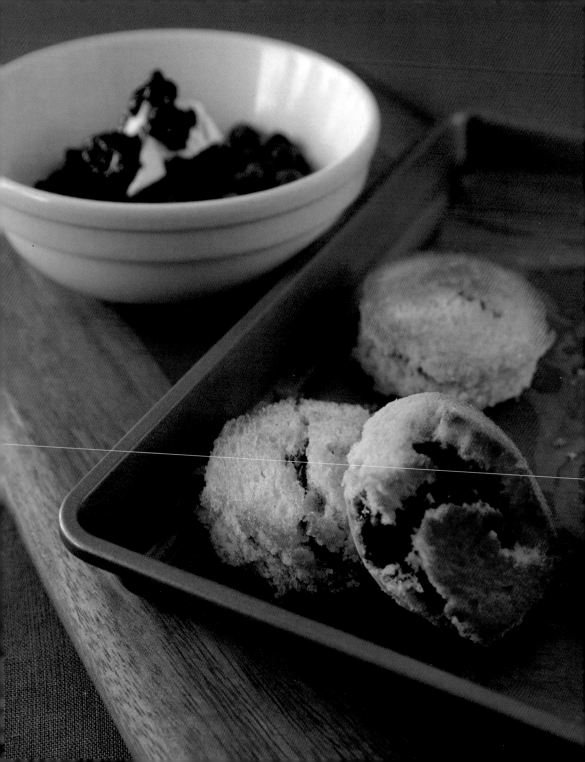

WHAT MAKES A GREAT PORTABLE?

Being based in Boulder, Colorado, means that we get to work with the top American cyclists on a regular basis. During the spring and summer of 2012, we hosted some training camps in Boulder, first to get riders ready for spring races, then the Tour de France, the London Olympic Games, and the World Championship road race. The recipes and ideas in this book were developed with feedback from the professional athletes we worked with during these camps and innumerable events like the Tour of California and USA Pro Challenge.

Some of these recipes in this cookbook may seem out of the ordinary, especially when compared to the standard fare of pre-packaged sports bars, blocks, and gels. From start to finish, we wanted to provide simple recipes that can make you feel good and perform better. Not only does portable food need to taste good, it needs to:

Pack in plenty of water to help with hydration and digestion ★ Provide enough energy, calories and carbs, to sustain an hour of effort ★ Fit into your jersey pocket or fuel belt ★ Unwrap easily and resist crumbling ★ Use ingredients that are easy to digest

If it can do all that, it's worth the effort.

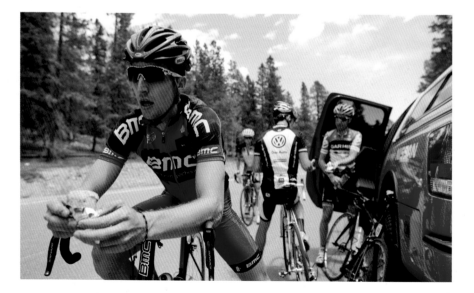

RULES TO RIDE BY

1 **Bigger makes for better texture and flavor.** All of our recipes are made with coarse salt and sugar. If you have to use table salt or fine sugars, start by adding half of the amount listed in the recipe, then adjust up to your liking.

2 **A little bit of sweetness goes a long way.** Use sugar to sweeten your portables and try to stick to unsweetened ingredients when the recipe calls for milk, yogurt, or coconut.

3 **Bold flavors are taken best sitting down.** When making ride or workout foods, use mild ingredients and keep the seasoning light. The same dishes can be more bold when cooking for boxed lunches or at home. The opposite is true for salt.

4 **Don't choke.** Whether you use a knife or a food processor, take care to mince or finely chop ingredients so they go down easy in the midst of a hard effort.

5 **There's no shortcutting sticky.** It's important to use fresh-cooked carbs in most of these recipes. The moisture is what holds the food together and helps it last longer once individually wrapped and stored.

COMMON FEED ZONE PORTABLES INGREDIENTS

Rice

We often use white rice with our athletes because it cooks faster, has a higher glycemic index (which can be good immediately after training), and is culturally what we're accustomed to. Brown rice is a fine substitute in most of the recipes (rice cakes being the exception).

Be careful about substituting. Calrose and jasmine rice are recommended in many cases and are always recommended for rice cakes. We also use basmati rice sometimes, but never for the rice cakes, as the rice won't stick together. Just don't try to use microwavable or instant rice for any recipe in this book. Why? Because the dishes won't taste very good, if they actually turn out, and because Biju and I will take it as a personal offense.

Recently, a lot of valid concern about arsenic in rice has emerged, especially from rice grown in very industrial areas such as midwestern regions along the Mississippi River. For this reason, we recommend a few things:

Try to purchase organic rice. ★ Use white polished rice that has the outer coating removed, which is the part of the rice grain that will retain the most contaminant. ★ Rinse your rice thoroughly at least a few times or until the water is mostly clear. Not only will cleaning the rice make it taste better, but it will help to wash away any chemicals.

Eggs

We use the entire egg, and lots of them. Eggs do contain quite a bit of cholesterol, and for the average American the conventional wisdom is that this may lead to an increase in blood cholesterol and thereby increase the risk of heart and peripheral vascular disease. A number of factors can affect the relationship between dietary and blood cholesterol—namely, physical activity and genetics. If you're not physically active, you might want to restrict yourself to averaging one or two eggs a day. If you have a family history of high cholesterol or know that you have high cholesterol, you might already know you need to restrict the amount of eggs in your diet.

The truth is, eggs are a very easy and convenient source of very high quality protein. Protein quality is graded on a scale, with a 1.0 being the highest grade of protein. The egg white is the only protein that scores a 1.0, and it is what all other proteins are effectively graded against. In addition, cholesterol is an essential back-

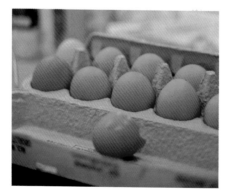

bone for all anabolic hormones in the body and is a vital nutrient. In the end, just as sugar alone is not going to give you diabetes, having cholesterol in your diet isn't going to give you a heart attack.

If you have concerns, talk to your doctor; in addition, get regular checkups and know your own body. The fact that we use eggs in our cookbook doesn't remove your responsibility, nor does it spell doomsday.

Salt

Sodium is one of the most important electrolytes in the human body. It controls the function of every cell in our body, propagating electrical signals through our nervous system and playing a vital role in fluid balance. We lose a lot of salt and electrolytes when we exercise—between 600 mg and 1,500 mg of sodium per liter of sweat, or about 300 to 750 mg of sodium per standard 500-ml bottle of sports drink. Most sports drinks don't contain enough sodium, and if we don't get enough sodium in our diets, then when we exercise, our function can deteriorate. In fact, we can become paradoxically more dehydrated by drinking water alone because the body increases urine output to maintain the concentration of sodium.

In addition to an inability to hold onto fluids, there is some interesting evidence showing that over time, we can slowly deplete the total sodium stored in the body as a result of heavy sweating during exercise. Normally, the total amount of sodium in the body is 1.3 grams per kilogram of

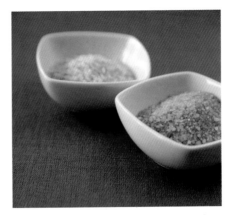

body weight, or 91 grams for a 70-kg (154-lb.) person. A 20 percent drop, equivalent to about 18 grams of sodium, in a 70-kg person can cause some real issues, including severe fatigue and all of the signs and symptoms associated with overreaching and overtraining syndrome. While most of us would be pretty hard pressed to lose that much salt in a single bout of exercise, it's conceivable that a little bit of loss each day during a hard stage race can create a deficit that results in real fatigue. With that in mind, if you know you are active and sweating a lot and you are craving salt, satiate that craving. It may help keep you from falling off the edge.

Of course, some individuals are salt-sensitive and can experience a dangerous rise in their blood pressure when they consume too much salt. If you know you feel really bloated and your blood pressure skyrockets when you add a lot of salt to your food, then do the rational thing and put the shaker down.

Most of the recipes in this book call for coarse salt, liquid amino acids, or low-sodium soy sauce. The latter two can be used interchangeably. If you are watching your sodium intake, try a spray version of the liquid amino acids or salt and add textured salt only after you finish cooking.

Sugar

Sugar is a vital energy source, especially for competitive cyclists. For example, in the Tour de France, simple sugars, especially in sports drinks, can make up the major-

ity of the calories consumed. Imagine if one of those athletes tried eating all of those calories in solid form. He would produce so much fecal matter that he literally would be sitting on the toilet for five hours the next day, rather than in his saddle. And while I concede most of us are not riding in the Tour, just because sugar is normally associated with nutritionally poor processed foods doesn't mean that it doesn't have a role in wholesome meals made from scratch or in sports drinks during exercise.

It's important to remember that most of the things that are ergogenic or performance enhancing during exercise can kill us when we are sitting on the couch. So if you aren't active, working hard, or sweating, keep the sugar at bay. Otherwise, realize that it can help when you are physically active and that everything works better in moderation.

You can use the following sugars interchangeably in most of our recipes: raw sugar, brown sugar, honey, and maple syrup. Brown sugar is the most affordable and accessible option. All of these are real sugars.

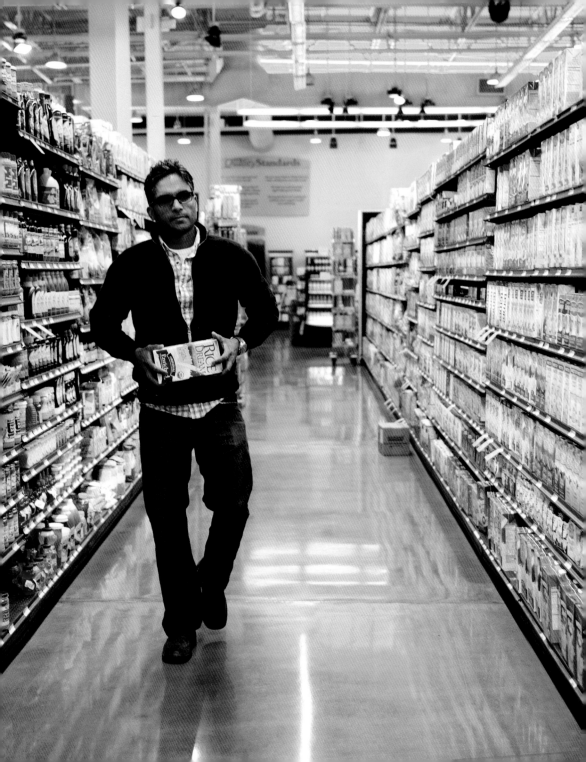

THE ATHLETE'S KITCHEN

IN THE FRIDGE

FRUITS

☆ Bananas
☆ Blueberries
☆ Dried fruit (currants, dates, raisins)
☆ Lemons
☆ Raspberries
☆ Strawberries

VEGETABLES

☆ Beets
☆ Carrots
☆ Celery
☆ Ginger
☆ Green onions/scallions
☆ Leeks
☆ Mushrooms
☆ Onions
☆ Peppers
☆ Potatoes
☆ Pumpkin
☆ Spinach
☆ Sweet potatoes
☆ Tomato
☆ Zucchini

FRESH HERBS

☆ Basil
☆ Cilantro
☆ Mint
☆ Parsley
☆ Tarragon
☆ Thyme

DAIRY

☆ Butter
☆ Cheese (cheddar, Swiss, parmesan, ricotta)
☆ Cream cheese
☆ Eggs
☆ Greek yogurt
☆ Milk (almond, coconut, dairy, or soy)

MEAT

☆ Bacon
☆ Beef
☆ Chicken
☆ Chicken sausage
☆ Deli meat
☆ Ham

IN THE PANTRY

BREAD

☆ Gluten-free bread
☆ Soft bread (buttermilk, potato, wheat)
☆ Soft bread rolls

FLOUR

☆ All-purpose flour
☆ Masa harina
☆ Mochi flour
☆ Potato flour
☆ Rice flour/ brown rice flour

GRAINS

☆ Grits
☆ Lentils
☆ Oats (old-fashioned rolled)
☆ Pasta
☆ Polenta
☆ Quinoa
☆ Rice (calrose, basmati, brown)

DRY GOODS

☆ Adzuki beans
☆ Baking powder
☆ Black beans
☆ Bouillon cubes
☆ Chocolate chips
☆ Coconut (unsweetened shredded)
☆ Coconut milk (canned)
☆ Instant idli mix
☆ Nuts (almonds, peanuts, pecans, walnuts)
☆ Potato flakes
☆ Salt (coarse)
☆ Sugar (raw, brown, etc.)
☆ Yeast (dry active)

CONDIMENTS

☆ Balsamic vinegar
☆ Canola oil
☆ Cocoa powder (unsweetened)
☆ Coconut oil
☆ Honey
☆ Ketchup
☆ Maple syrup
☆ Molasses
☆ Nut butter
☆ Almond butter
☆ Peanut butter
☆ Olive oil

☆ Preserves
☆ Tomato paste
☆ Soy sauce (low-sodium)
☆ Vinegar (apple cider, red wine)

SPICES

☆ Celery salt
☆ Chili powder
☆ Cinnamon
☆ Cream of tartar
☆ Crystallized ginger
☆ Cumin
☆ Curry powder
☆ Garlic powder
☆ Old Bay seasoning
☆ Onion powder
☆ Paprika
☆ Vanilla extract

EQUIPMENT

APPLIANCES

☆ Food processor (small, inexpensive)
☆ Rice cooker

OPTIONAL

☆ Electric mixer
☆ Juicer
☆ Waffle iron

FOR COOKING & BAKING

☆ 4.5–6 quart large pot
☆ 8" or 9" square baking pan
☆ 9" × 12" rimmed baking pan
☆ Large sauté pan
☆ Muffin tin

FOR PREP

☆ Cutting board
☆ Knives of assorted sizes
☆ Large mixing bowl
☆ Measuring cups and spoons
☆ Rolling pin
☆ Spatula and mixing spoons
☆ Strainer

FOR PACKAGING

☆ Airtight storage containers
☆ Paper foil
☆ Plastic wrap
☆ Sharp knife
☆ Ziplock bags

TIP Discount retailers such as T.J. Maxx and Ross often have good kitchen supplies at an affordable price.

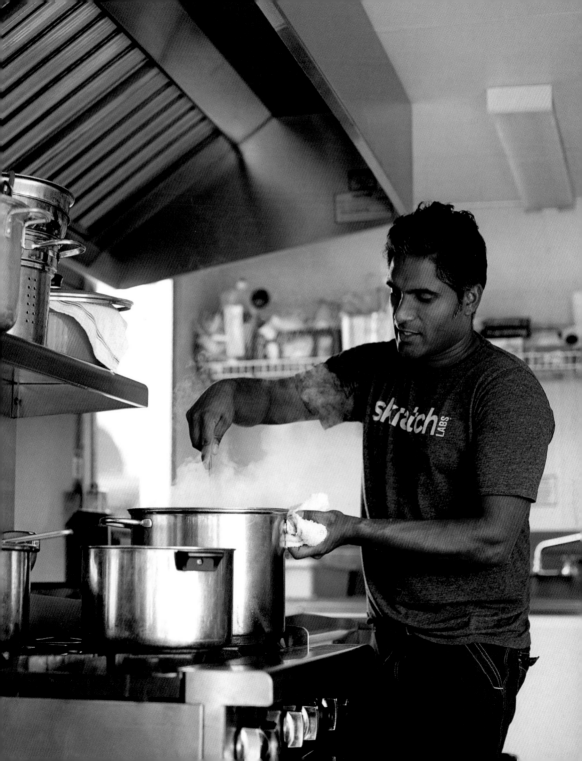

CUTTING **PAPER FOIL**

Paper foil makes the perfect wrapper for portables because it doesn't stick to the food. Rather than cutting individual sheets as you need them, here's a quick way to have a stack of paper foil ready for your next batch of portables.

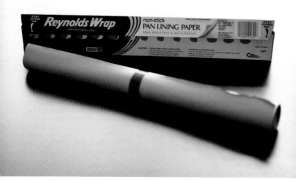

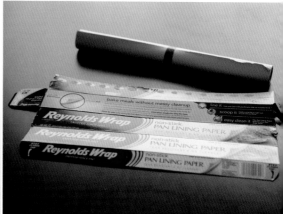

You can find paper foil at your local grocery store. (We use the Reynolds Wrap brand, which they call "nonstick pan lining paper.")

★ Remove the roll of paper foil and flatten the paperboard box.

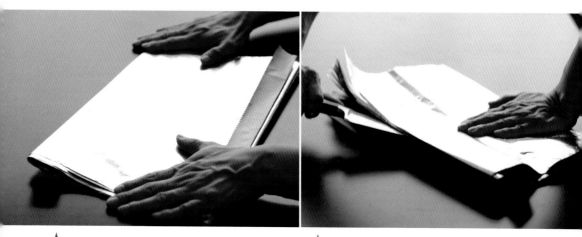

★ Firmly press the folded edges on each side to create a nice crease. Pull out the paperboard.

★ Use a sharp knife to cut along one side of the paper foil. Repeat on the other side. Divide into two long paper stacks.

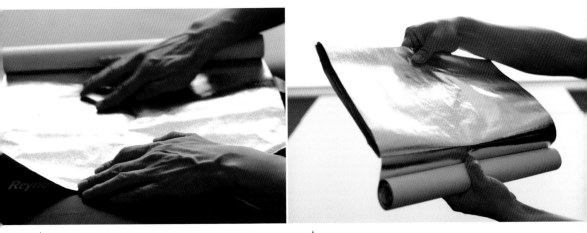

⭐ 2 Line up the edge of the paper foil with the edge of the flattened paperboard.

⭐ 3 Wrap the roll around the paperboard, keeping it snug around the edges, until you reach the end of the roll.

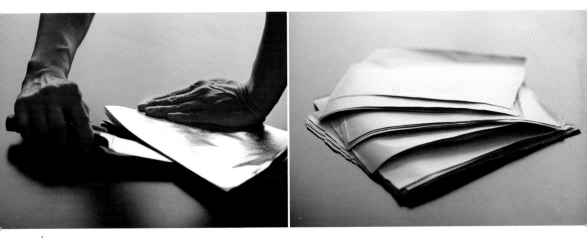

⭐ Fold one of the stacks of paper in half, making a sheet that is roughly 9" × 7". Firmly press the folded edge to create a nice crease. Use the knife to cut along the fold. Repeat with the second stack.

Now you are ready to wrap up portables. (See Wrap It Up, page 62.)

WRAP IT UP

A well-wrapped portable will give you easy access to fresh food when you need it most. This method works well for most any portable snack, from rice cakes to kugel.

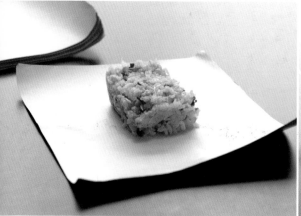 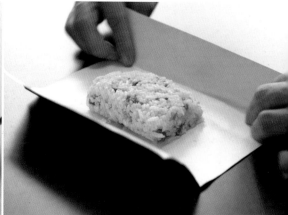

⭐ Cut your food item roughly the size and shape of a brownie. Place the food in the center of a square sheet of paper foil (roughly 8 inches square), with the parchment side up.

⭐ Fold in the two sides of paper foil along the long edge of the rice cake with the edges overlapping.

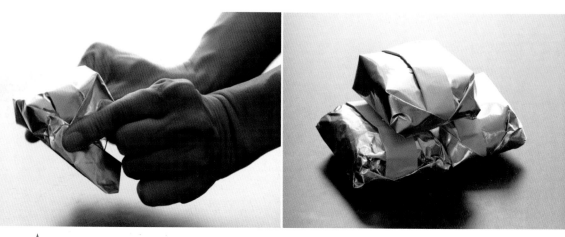

⭐ Tuck the triangular tabs at each end underneath the wrapped edges.

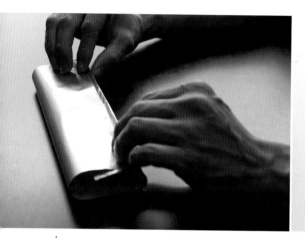

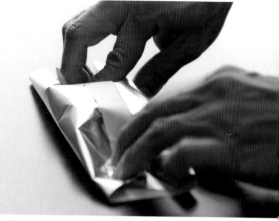

★3 Make a crease on the outside edge of the top layer of foil. This will help you open the wrapper and create a little pocket to help you hold the food without getting your hands dirty.

★4 Fold the two open sides of the foil into triangle tabs as you would to wrap a gift.

TIP Portables will keep fresh longer if you individually wrap them. Cut and wrap cooled slices and store them in the fridge in a sealed plastic bag. **GRAB AND GO!**

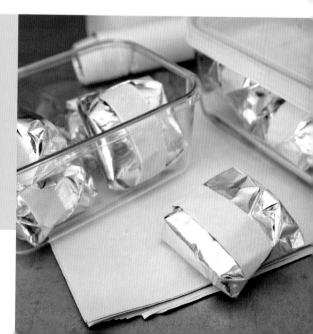

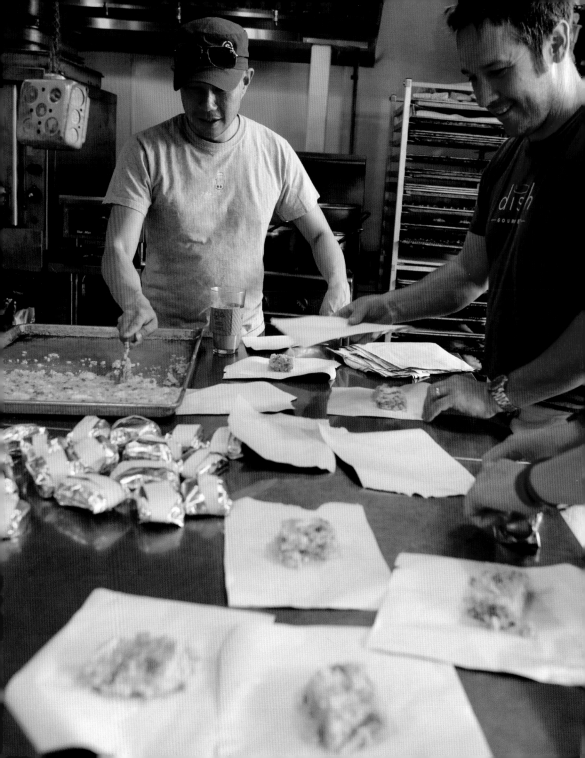

RICE CAKES

A hearty rice cake is the perfect on-the-go food, offering the comfort and flavor of a great meal. Rice cakes have become a staple in the pro peloton.

We had the opportunity to direct the menu for the USA Pro Challenge, a domestic stage race in our home state of Colorado. Soigneurs lined up shoulder to shoulder to wrap rice cakes for their teams. Cyclists love Allen's original recipe with eggs and bacon, which is undeniably a great portable for race day.

Since the publication of *The Feed Zone Cookbook*, we've been experimenting with some other flavors, and we are confident that you will find something new to pack into your jersey pocket or tuck away for whatever the day holds.

Layered rice cakes are another new addition. Last night's leftover dinner can often make a great filler for a sticky rice sandwich, so try out some of your favorites.

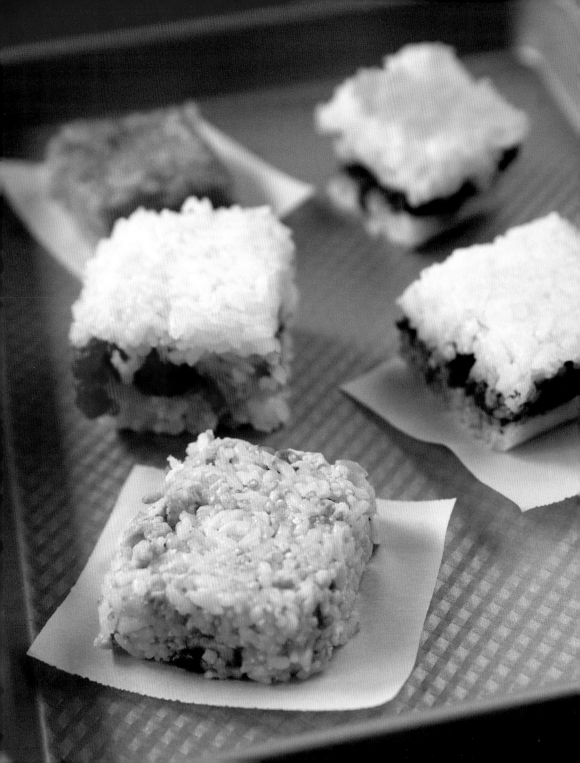

V VEGETARIAN   G GLUTEN-FREE

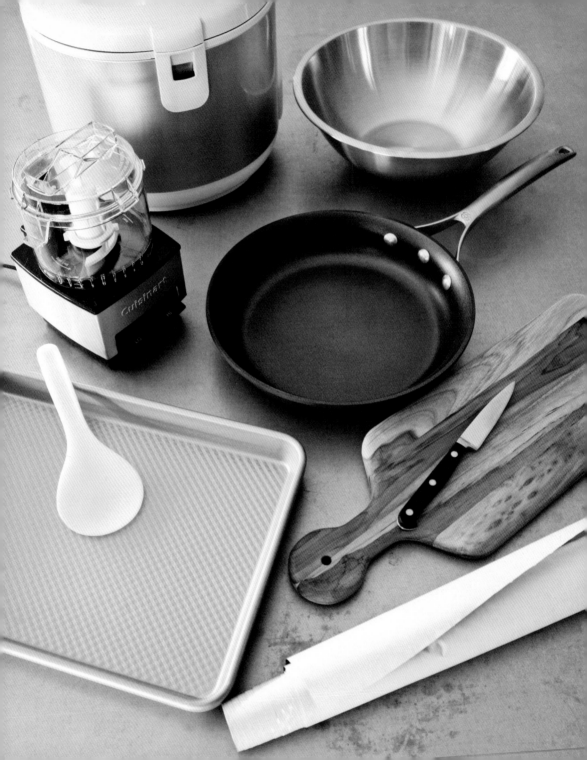

EQUIPMENT

☆ Rice cooker / Large saucepan

☆ Small food processor / Knife and cutting board

☆ Large sauté pan (for rice cakes with cooked ingredients)

☆ Large mixing bowl

☆ 9" × 12" rimmed baking pan

☆ Rice paddle or smooth rubber spatula

☆ Sharp knife

☆ Paper foil for wrapping

★ We're confident that you will get your money's worth out of an inexpensive **PANASONIC RICE COOKER**. But until you make the leap, here's a simple stovetop method for cooking sticky rice:

Combine calrose (medium-grain "sticky") rice, water, and a dash of salt in a large saucepan. Bring rice to a low rolling boil, cover, and cook over low heat until the water has evaporated, about 10 minutes. Turn heat off and leave covered for another 10 minutes.

HOW TO MAKE PERFECT STICKY RICE

Fresh-cooked rice is the essential ingredient in rice cakes because the rice is stickier when it's warm, helping the cake hold together.

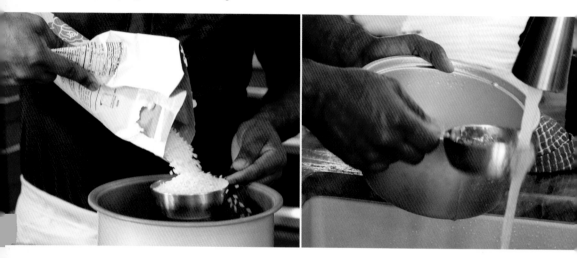

When making rice cakes, the texture will vary based on how much moisture is in your rice and the proportions of rice to wet ingredients. Go slowly so you can find the magical combination of "stickiness" and flavor. If your rice cakes are a little dry, try ★ rinsing the rice under cool water before cooking, or ★ adding more water to the rice before cooking.

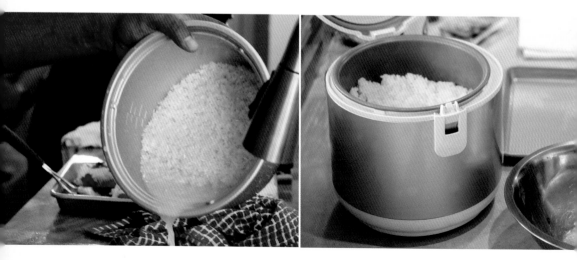

Many of our portable recipes call for uncooked "sticky" rice. **CALROSE RICE**, a strain of medium-grain rice common in Asian cooking, is widely available. This variety cooks fast (in 20 minutes or less in most rice cookers), retains a nutty flavor, and is just sticky enough to hold our cakes together. Any "sushi rice" variety should work well for making portables.

THE DENVER RICE CAKE

3 cups uncooked sticky rice

4½ cups water

¼ cup chopped fresh tomato

1 tablespoon minced bell pepper

¼ cup diced ham

2 tablespoons minced onion

6 eggs, lightly beaten

¼ cup grated cheddar cheese

OPTIONAL ADDITIONS

½ teaspoon celery salt

Sriracha sauce to taste

Combine rice, water, and a dash of salt in a rice cooker and let cook.

Bring a sauté pan to medium-high heat with just enough oil to coat bottom of the pan. Add tomatoes, bell peppers, ham, and onions. Cook mixture until onions are translucent.

Pour in eggs and cook for just a few minutes, until eggs are almost dry and all ingredients are incorporated well. Remove from heat.

Add any optional additions here.

Combine rice with cooked ingredients. Evenly spread into a 9" × 12" baking pan and sprinkle with cheese.

Stir in the cheese here if you prefer.

Let set up for a few minutes, then cut into squares and wrap.

TIP If you are a **VEGETARIAN**, substitute any variety of cooked or canned beans for the ham. Fully drain all liquid, then mash the beans before mixing into the rice cake mixture.

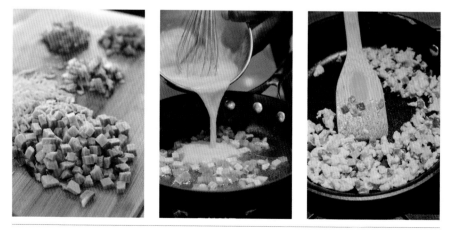

PER SERVING› Energy 185 cal, **Fat** 3 g, **Sodium** 78 mg, **Carbs** 31 g, **Fiber** 1 g, **Protein** 6 g, **Water** 70%
Nutrition facts for optional additions can be found in Appendix B.

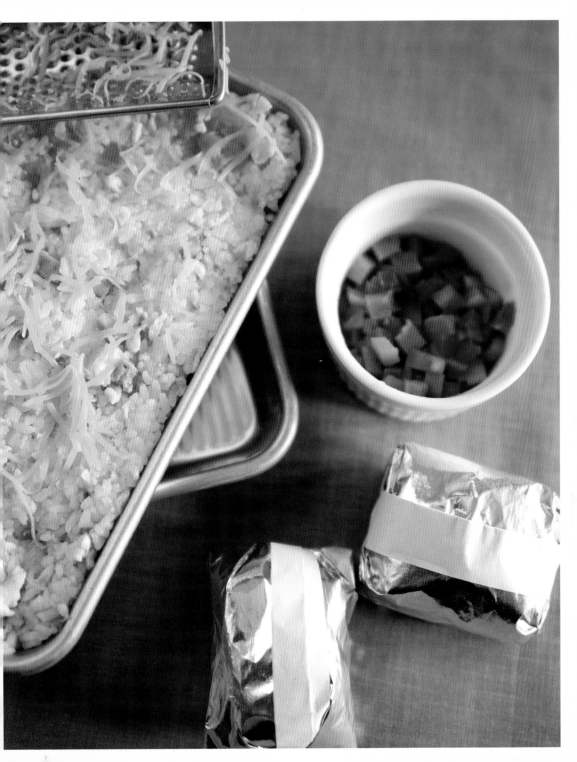

RED LENTIL RICE CAKES

1 cup uncooked red lentils

2 cups uncooked sticky rice

4½ cups water

1 tablespoon minced onion

1½ teaspoons minced jalapeno pepper

1 teaspoon sweet paprika

1½ teaspoons tomato paste

¼ cup plain Greek yogurt

coarse salt and pepper to taste

OPTIONAL ADDITIONS

½ cup diced tomato (add to pan with onion and pepper)

1 teaspoon chopped scallions

1 tablespoon minced cilantro or parsley

1 teaspoon Tabasco

Rinse lentils in cold water, then drain. Combine lentils, rice, water, and a dash of salt in rice cooker and let cook.

While rice and lentils are cooking, bring sauté pan to medium-high heat with just enough oil to coat bottom of pan, and lightly cook the onions and peppers. Sprinkle in paprika while continuing to stir the mixture. If needed, add more oil to keep the mixture from sticking.

Stir in tomato paste while scraping pan, then turn heat to low and add yogurt. Mix thoroughly and remove from heat.

When the rice and lentils are finished cooking (the lentils will be a pale yellow), add to sautéed vegetables and yogurt mixture. Adjust salt to taste. Evenly spread mixture into a 9" × 12" baking pan.

Add any optional additions here.

Let set up for a few minutes, then cut into squares and wrap.

PER SERVING› **Energy** 150 cal, **Fat** 1 g, **Sodium** 110 mg, **Carbs** 30 g, **Fiber** 2 g, **Protein** 5 g, **Water** 67%
Nutrition facts for optional additions can be found in Appendix B.

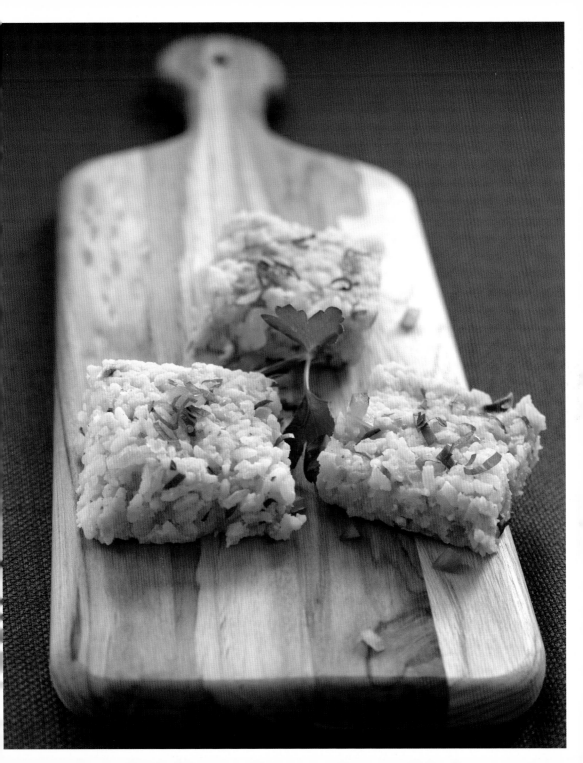

CARBOHYDRATES COUNT

If you take a look at nutrition facts for different sources of carbohydrates, you can see why white rice is the star ingredient in portable foods. High in calories and low in fiber, rice is an efficient fuel. Potatoes, on the other hand, are lower in calories per weight but higher in water content. Quinoa is a good source of protein. Fiber is great for your diet but easier to manage when you are not riding, so incorporate lentils in your postworkout portables. Try different carbohydrate sources to find the balance of carbohydrate, fiber, and protein that works best for you.

COOKED INGREDIENT	MEASURE	ENERGY (CAL)	FAT (G)	SODIUM (MG)	CARB (G)	FIBER (G)	PROTEIN (G)	WATER (%)
Lentils, red	1 cup	230	1	4	40	16	18	70
Oats, old-fashioned rolled	1 cup	166	4	9	32	4	6	84
Pasta, orzo	1 cup	200	1	–	42	2	7	72
Potato	1 medium	145	–	8	34	2	3	76
Sweet Potato	1 medium	103	–	41	24	4	2	75
Quinoa	1 cup	222	4	13	39	5	8	71
Rice, white sticky/calrose	1 cup	242	–	–	53	1	4	69
Rice, brown	1 cup	218	2	2	46	4	5	73

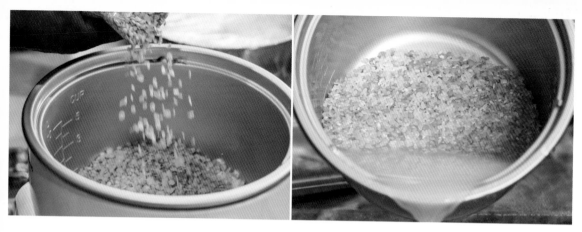

MAKING THE MOST OF YOUR RICE COOKER

By mixing in another carbohydrate with your rice, you can change up the texture or flavor of different portables. Simply add the lentils, quinoa, or oats along with the rice and let the rice cooker do the rest.

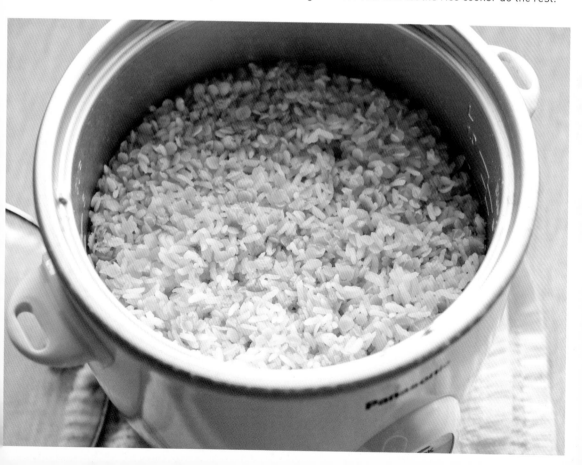

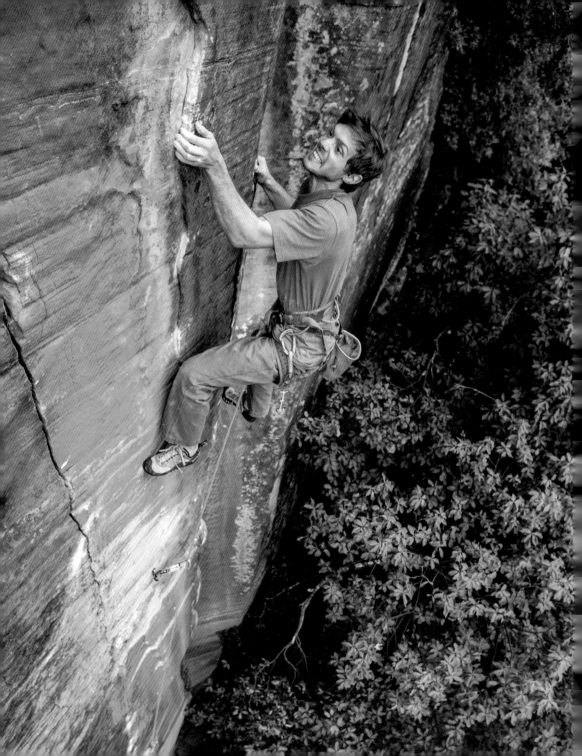

★ ★ ★

"As a professional rock climber, I spend many full days in the mountains pushing my physical and mental limits. For many years my daily nutrition was similar to most outdoor adventure athletes: extremely processed bars and gels by day and simple pre-packaged meals by night.

"After being introduced to *The Feed Zone*, I began to realize there was another way to eat that actually nourished me as an athlete. I didn't have to live off of processed bars, which dehydrated me and upset my stomach.

"I started trying recipe after recipe and fell in love with making (and eating) rice cakes. I found they were the perfect snack to help me sustain a full day of climbing. It was great to actually be eating real food throughout the day."

MATT SEGAL
MEMBER OF THE NORTH FACE ATHLETE TEAM
FIRST ASCENT OF THE IRON MONKEY 5.14R, ELDORADO CANYON, CO
FIRST ASCENT OF ORANGUTAN OVERHANG 5.14, INDEPENDENCE PASS, CO

MASALA CHICKEN RICE CAKES

Curry wins over many a professional cyclist. Both savory and sweet, curry is a pleasant change of pace and readily available throughout Europe, from currywurst in Germany to curry ketchup on frites in Belgium and the Netherlands. Curry doesn't have to be complicated to taste great. Try out our Curry Potato & Chicken Pies (page 124) and judge for yourself.

3 cups uncooked sticky rice

4½ cups water

2 tablespoons minced onion

1 tablespoon minced jalapeno pepper

1 tablespoon mild curry powder

¼ cup tomato sauce or ketchup

8 ounces ground chicken

½ cup plain Greek yogurt

coarse salt and pepper to taste

OPTIONAL ADDITIONS

more curry powder

½ cup diced tomato (add to pan with onion and pepper)

1 teaspoon minced fresh ginger

1 teaspoon minced cilantro

You can substitute boneless, skinless chicken breast for ground chicken.

Combine rice, water, and a dash of salt in a rice cooker and let cook.

While rice is cooking, bring a sauté pan to medium-high heat with just enough oil to coat bottom of the pan.

If using chicken breast, add here.

Cook onions and peppers until the onions become translucent.

Add the curry powder while continually scraping the pan. If needed, add more oil to keep the mixture from sticking. Stir in the tomato sauce while still scraping pan.

Add chicken and cook until it is cooked through and begins to brown, about 5 minutes. Reduce heat to low and stir in yogurt. Mix thoroughly and remove from heat.

When the rice is finished cooking, add it to the chicken and vegetables. Add salt to taste and evenly spread into a 9" × 12" baking pan.

Add any optional additions here.

Let set up for a few minutes, then cut into squares and wrap.

TIP For a bigger flavor punch, add more CURRY POWDER (3–4 tablespoons total). Keep the flavor mild for ride food.

PER SERVING › Energy 179 cal, Fat 2 g, Sodium 66 mg, Carbs 33 g, Fiber 1 g, Protein 6 g, Water 66%
Nutrition facts for optional additions can be found in Appendix B.

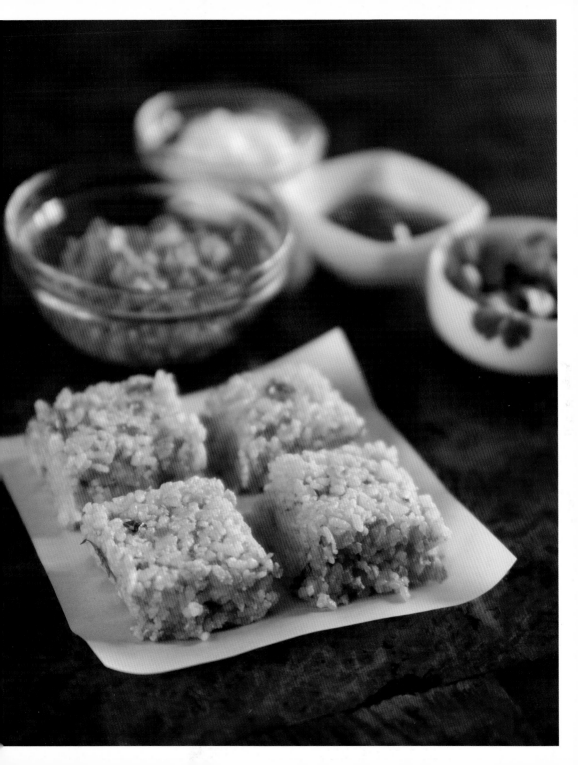

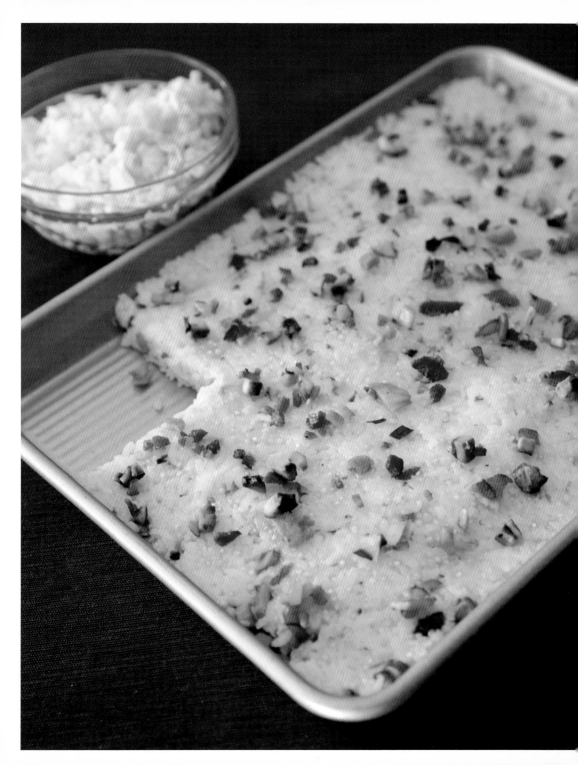

SWISS RICE CAKES

2 cups uncooked sticky rice

1 cup quinoa

4½ cups water

4 ounces chopped bacon

2 tablespoons onion, minced

6 eggs, lightly beaten (optional)

½ cup sliced mushrooms

¼ cup shredded Swiss or
Emmentaler cheese

1 tablespoon minced
fresh tarragon

coarse salt and pepper to taste

OPTIONAL ADDITIONS

½ teaspoon celery salt

Tabasco to taste

*Dry tarragon works nicely—
reduce to just ½ teaspoon to avoid
overpowering the other flavors.*

Combine rice, quinoa, water, and a dash of salt in a rice cooker and let cook.

While the rice is cooking, place the bacon (if using) in a sauté pan and cook over medium-high heat. Transfer cooked bacon to a paper towel to cool. Drain the bacon fat from the pan, leaving just enough to sauté the onions. If you are not using bacon, add a small amount of oil to the pan.

Sauté the onions until translucent, then add mushrooms and cook until tender. Remove from heat and stir in the cooked bacon.

If using eggs, add after the onions cook.

When the rice is finished cooking, add it to the cooked ingredients and stir in the cheese and tarragon. Once all ingredients are incorporated, evenly spread the mixture into a 9" × 12" baking pan.

Add any optional additions here.

Let set up for a few minutes, then cut into squares and wrap.

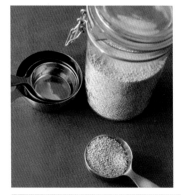

Pack some protein into your rice cakes with **QUINOA**. Combine 2 cups of rice and 1 cup of quinoa in the rice cooker. Adding lentils to rice cakes works the same way.

PER SERVING› Energy 177 cal, **Fat** 5 g, **Sodium** 76 mg, **Carbs** 28 g, **Fiber** 1 g, **Protein** 5 g, **Water** 68%
Nutrition facts for optional additions can be found in Appendix B.

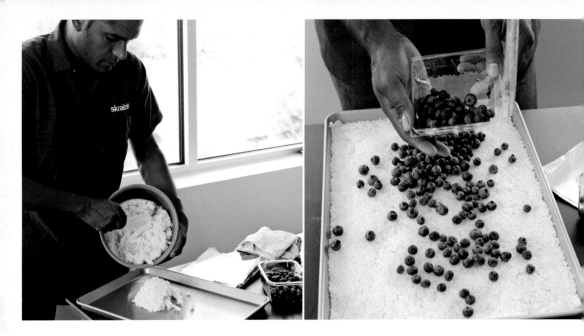

LAYERED RICE CAKES

Seasoning your rice is an important step in making layered rice cakes. For **SAVORY** layered rice cakes, season with salt—liquid aminos or low-sodium soy sauce are good options too. For **SWEET** layered rice cakes, add canned coconut milk or sugar and balance out the sweetness with a zing of fresh citrus. Find your own perfect formula for texture and flavor.

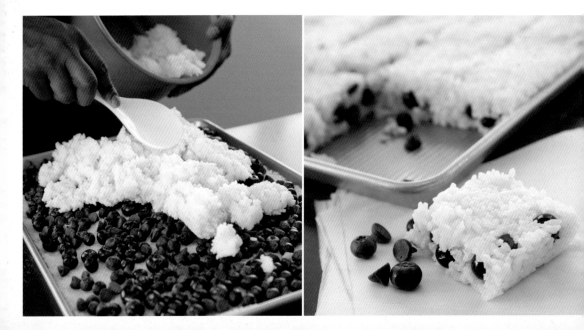

★ ★ ★

"I never bonk when I have rice cakes in my pocket—anything with coconut is my favorite. I like to make a fresh batch at the start of the week using whatever I have in my kitchen, so I have my ride food taken care of for a few days."

EVELYN STEVENS
1ST, FLÈCHE WALLONNE
SILVER MEDALIST, UCI WORLD
CHAMPIONSHIPS, TIME TRIAL
2-TIME NATIONAL TIME TRIAL CHAMPION

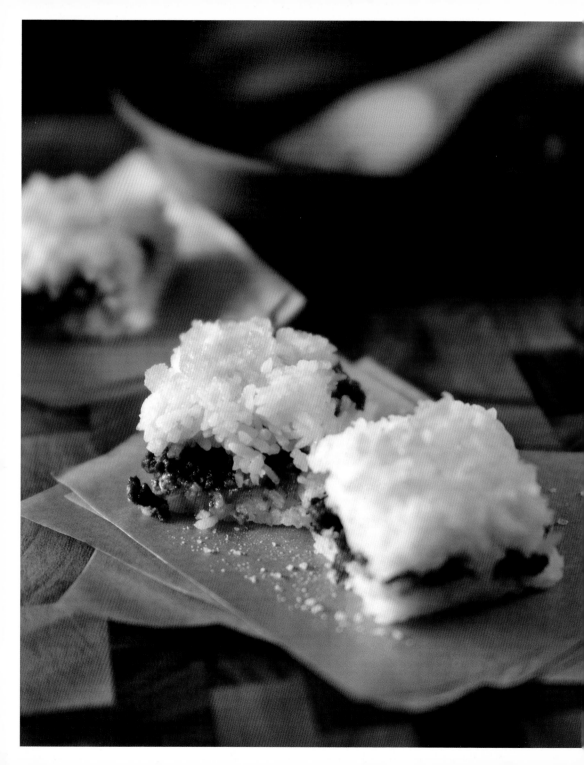

SPICED BEEF & ONION RICE CAKES

3 cups uncooked sticky rice

4½ cups water

8 ounces lean ground beef

2 tablespoons minced onion

½ cup molasses

1 tablespoon low-sodium soy sauce

1 tablespoon minced fresh ginger

1 teaspoon ground cinnamon

1 tablespoon chopped crystallized ginger

OPTIONAL ADDITIONS
(1 tablespoon of each)

grated parmesan

cilantro, minced

celery salt

balsamic vinegar

Beef minced in a small food processor can be used in place of ground beef.

Combine rice, water, and a dash of salt in a rice cooker and let cook.

While the rice is cooking, brown meat in a sauté pan over medium-high heat. Add onions and cook until they are translucent. Drain any excess fat.

Reduce heat to medium, then add molasses and soy sauce to the beef and onions. Cook for 2–3 minutes to incorporate liquids. Mix in the fresh ← ginger and cinnamon before removing from heat.

Once the rice has mostly cooled, season it to taste. *Add any* Transfer half of the rice into a 9" × 12" baking pan *optional* and press flat with a rice paddle. Add the beef *additions* mixture, spreading evenly. *here.*

Gently press the remaining rice on top to create the second layer. Top with coarsely chopped crystallized ginger.

Let set up for a few minutes, then cut into squares and wrap.

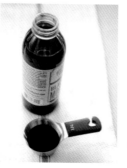

MOLASSES has a complex, earthy taste that people are drawn to. Look for unsulfured blackstrap molasses, which is a great source of manganese and iron.

PER SERVING› Energy 198 cal, Fat 1 g, **Sodium** 60 mg, **Carbs** 40 g, **Fiber** 1 g, **Protein** 6 g, **Water** 65%
Nutrition facts for optional additions can be found in Appendix B.

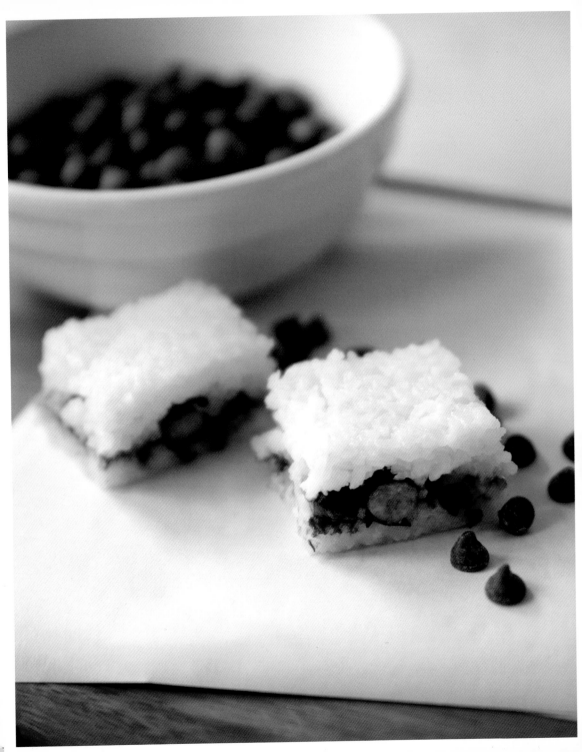

BLUEBERRY & CHOCOLATE COCONUT RICE CAKES

3 cups uncooked sticky rice

4½ cups water

¾ cup canned coconut milk

¼ cup raw sugar

juice of 1 lemon or other citrus (~3 tablespoons)

1½ teaspoons coarse salt, or to taste

6 ounces semisweet chocolate chips (half of a regular bag)

1 pint fresh blueberries

Combine rice, water, and a dash of salt in a rice cooker and let cook.

When the rice is finished cooking, transfer it to a large bowl and add coconut milk. Begin seasoning the rice with the sugar. The mixture should be slightly sweet to your palate (sometimes we use up to ½ cup of sugar). Squeeze in the lemon juice gradually, giving the mixture just a little bit of bite. Stir the rice mixture thoroughly and add salt to taste.

Once the rice has mostly cooled, spread half of the mixture into a 9" × 12" baking pan and press flat with a rice paddle. Then sprinkle the chocolate chips and berries evenly atop the rice. Gently press the remaining rice onto the berries and chocolate to create the second layer.

Let set up for a few minutes, then cut into squares and wrap.

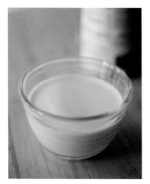

Canned **COCONUT MILK** is thicker and creamier than the coconut milk found in the refrigerated section of your grocery store.

PER SERVING› Energy 249 cal, **Fat** 6 g, **Sodium** 194 mg, **Carbs** 45 g, **Fiber** 2 g, **Protein** 4 g, **Water** 65%

RASPBERRY & MINT RICE CAKES

3 cups uncooked sticky rice

4½ cups water

½ cup cane sugar
(or your favorite sweetener)

juice of 1 lemon or other citrus
(~3 tablespoons)

1 pint fresh raspberries

2 tablespoons fresh
mint leaves, minced

OPTIONAL ADDITIONS

1 teaspoon vanilla extract

1 teaspoon honey

1 teaspoon minced fresh ginger

1 tablespoon unsweetened
shredded coconut

Combine rice, water, and a dash of salt in a rice cooker and let cook.

When the rice is finished cooking, transfer it to a large bowl and add sugar and lemon juice. Mix thoroughly. The mixture should be slightly sweet with a little bite from the fresh-squeezed citrus.

Add any optional additions here.

Spread half of the rice mixture onto a 9" × 12" baking pan, using a rice paddle to gently press the rice into the pan. Top with berries and sprinkle minced mint leaves evenly.

Finish by gently layering remaining rice over the top of the berries and mint.

Let set up for a few minutes, then cut into squares and wrap.

TIP You can substitute any **BERRY** for the raspberries, but use only fresh!

PER SERVING› Energy 176 cal, **Fat** 0 g, **Sodium** 10 mg, **Carbs** 40 g, **Fiber** 2 g, **Protein** 3 g, **Water** 68%
Nutrition facts for optional additions can be found in Appendix B.

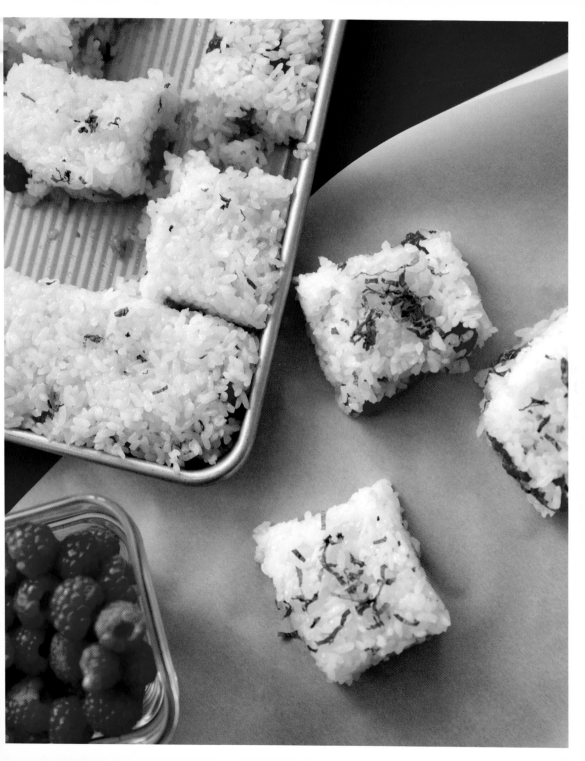

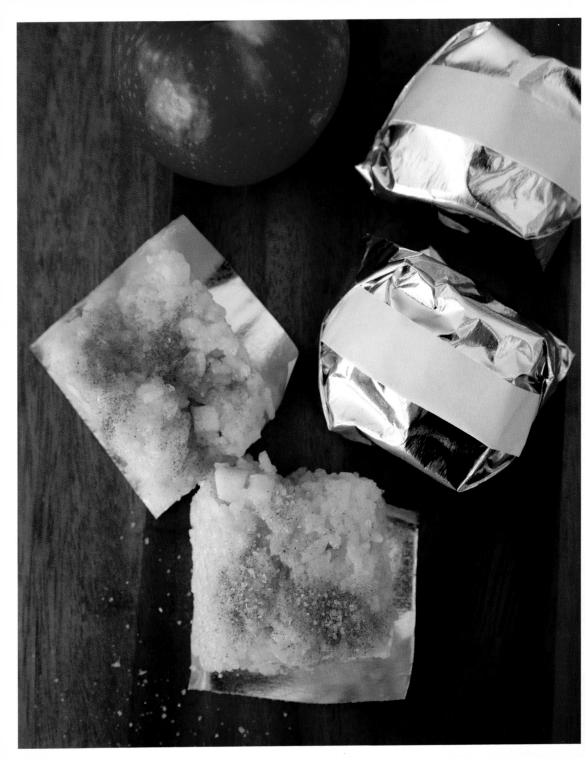

CINNAMON APPLE RICE CAKES

3 cups uncooked sticky rice

4½ cups water

1 apple, peeled and minced

2 tablespoons raw sugar

juice of 1 lemon
(~3 tablespoons)

TOP WITH

2 tablespoons raw sugar

2 teaspoons ground cinnamon

1 teaspoon coarse salt

Combine rice, water, and a dash of salt in a rice cooker and let cook.

When the rice is finished cooking, transfer it to a large bowl and add the apple, sugar, and lemon juice.

Once all ingredients are incorporated, adjust seasoning to taste. Evenly spread the mixture into a 9" × 12" baking pan and top with a sprinkling of cinnamon sugar and coarse salt.

Let set up for a few minutes, then cut into squares and wrap.

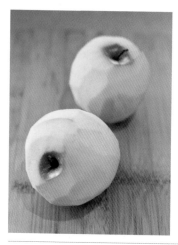

A firm, **TART APPLE** like Granny Smith will give these rice cakes a balanced flavor and texture.

PER SERVING › Energy 159 cal, **Fat** 0 g, **Sodium** 174 mg, **Carbs** 36 g, **Fiber** 1 g, **Protein** 3 g, **Water** 68%

PB&J RICE CAKES

3 cups uncooked sticky rice

4½ cups water

1 cup old-fashioned peanut butter

1 cup of your favorite fruit preserves (or your favorite sweetener)

Combine rice, water, and a dash of salt in a rice cooker and let cook.

When the rice is finished cooking, spread half of it onto a 9" × 12" baking pan, using a rice paddle to gently press the rice into the pan.

Use a rubber spatula to evenly spread the peanut butter over the rice, then place several dollops of preserves evenly atop the peanut butter. (When you add the top layer of rice, the jam will spread.)

Finish by gently pressing the remaining rice over the top.

Let set up for a few minutes, then cut into squares and wrap.

TIP To make a small batch of PB&J cakes using leftover rice: *While the rice is still warm*, press it into a pan. Spread peanut butter on one side and preserves on the other. Cut in half and use a spatula to flip one side, positioning the sticky sides together.

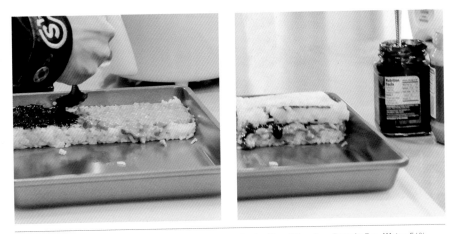

PER SERVING› Energy 301 cal, **Fat** 9 g, **Sodium** 95 mg, **Carbs** 49 g, **Fiber** 2 g, **Protein** 7 g, **Water** 56%

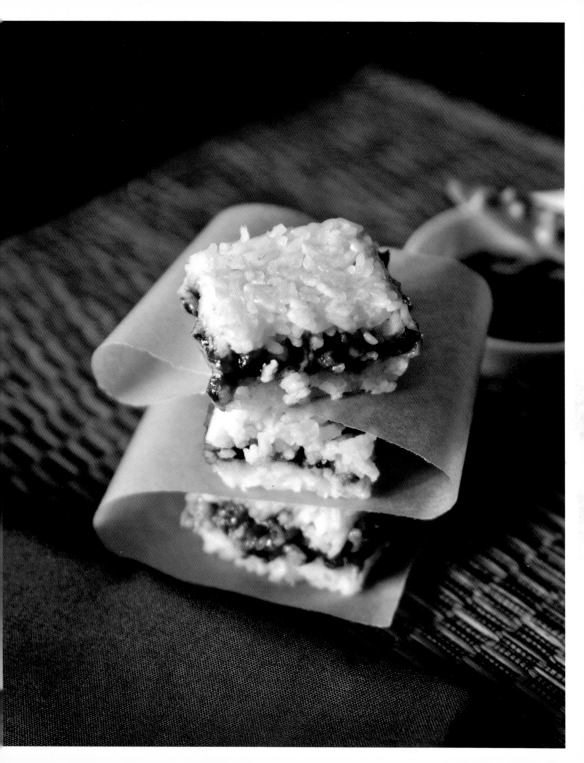

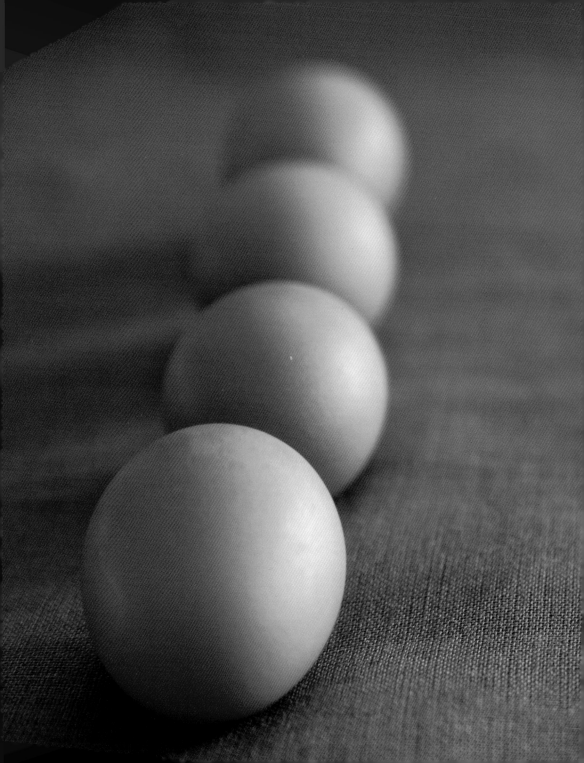

BAKED EGGS

In our experience, eggs are the peloton's favorite source of protein. It's as much about what is practical as it is about taste. Whether you are at home or on the road, eggs are affordable and easy to find.

When we are in the trailer cooking for athletes, we might need to serve up 50 eggs all at once. Muffin tins are a quick, efficient way to cook dozens of eggs to perfection.

Make a few eggs for your pre-ride meal and stock some extras in the fridge for snacks and tasty additions to sandwiches or salads.

V VEGETARIAN   **G** GLUTEN-FREE

FUSS-FREE COOKING WITH MUFFIN TINS

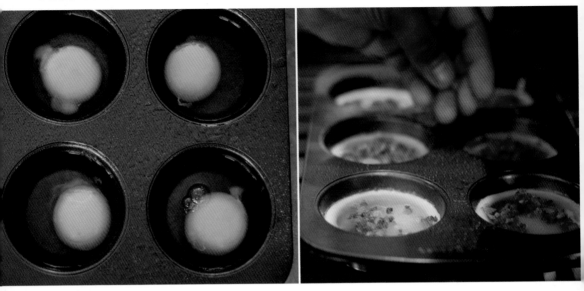

Pull the eggs out of the oven just before they fully set up. They will finish cooking in the pan.

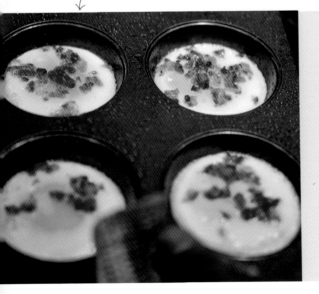

TIP Even with nonstick cooking spray, getting portables out of muffin tins can be difficult. Use a disposable knife— the hot pan helps the knife to easily slide around the edge of the muffin form and gently pull out the food inside.

> ★ ★ ★
>
> "The food that allows you to perform your best is really simple and easy to make. I've trained my stomach to handle a variety of food and flavors, especially on long rides. I love eggs and anything spicy."
>
> **TIMMY DUGGAN**
> *USPRO NATIONAL CHAMPION*
> *OLYMPIAN, ROAD RACING*

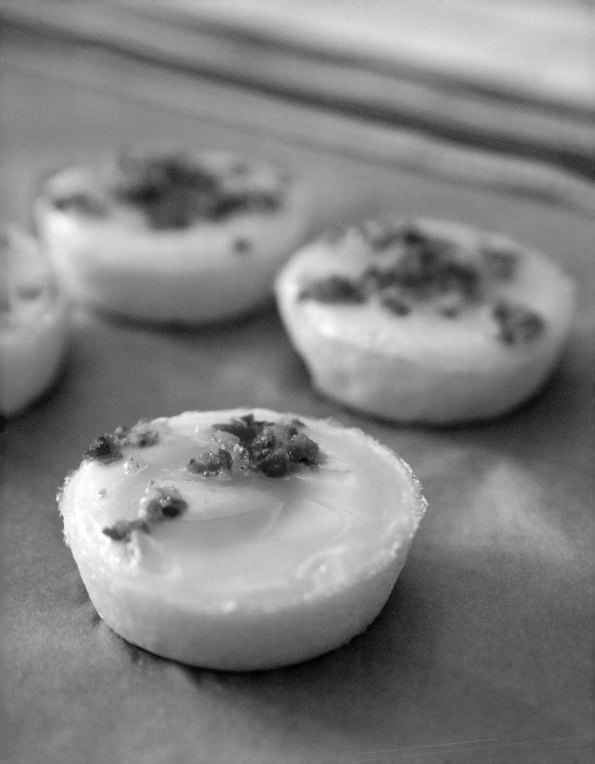

BASIC BAKED EGGS

6 eggs

COOKED 2 tablespoons
chopped cooked bacon

OPTIONAL ADDITIONS
¼ cup grated parmesan

salt and pepper

Heat oven to 350 degrees. Thoroughly coat six cups of a standard nonstick muffin tin with cooking spray.

Carefully crack one egg into each muffin form. Position pan on the middle rack of the oven. To evenly cook the eggs, rotate the pan after 5–6 minutes, or when the eggs begin to turn white.

Bake until the whites set and the yolks look partially set (about 10–15 minutes total). Remove from the oven; the eggs will continue to cook while resting. Sprinkle with bacon or salt and pepper to taste.

Add cheese here if using.

While the eggs are resting, use a plastic knife to loosen them from the edge of the pan. Let cool to the touch before wrapping. Store extras in the refrigerator.

TIP Press soft bread slices into a muffin tin to make a **QUICK CRUST** for baked eggs (see page 137). Increase baking time to 20–25 minutes. The bread will get crusty on the edges.

PER SERVING› **Energy** 80 cal, **Fat** 6 g, **Sodium** 178 mg, **Carbs** 0 g, **Fiber** 0 g, **Protein** 7 g, **Water** 63%
Nutrition facts for optional additions can be found in Appendix B.

Begin with fresh, whole foods that come in their own wrapper with as many of their parts intact as possible—foods that are *minimally processed, grown locally and preferably organically.*

STACK IT

Stack your egg on some carbs for a more filling portable before or after your workout›
Sweet potato/potato ★ Sticky rice ★ Bread/quick crust ★ Sweet polenta ★ Pumpkin

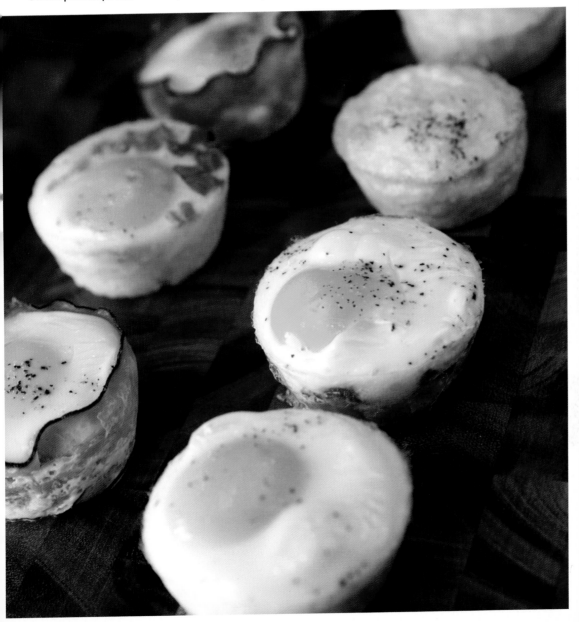

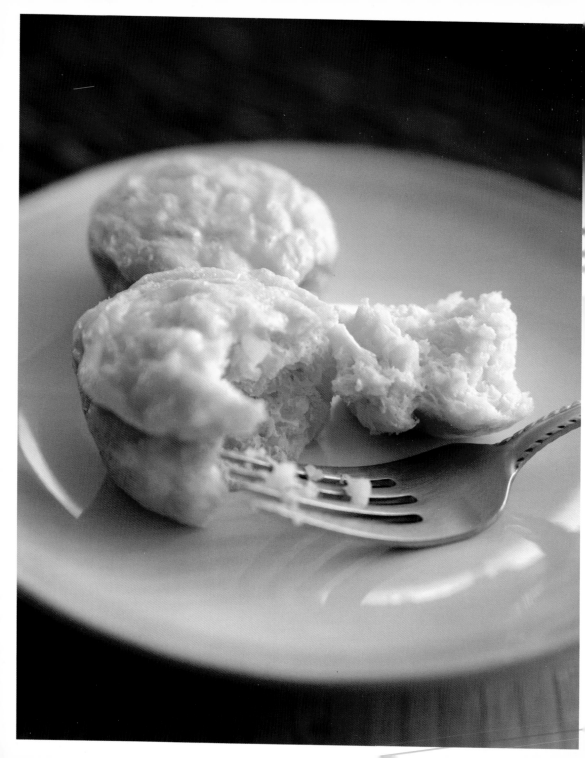

RICE SOUFFLÉ

4 eggs + 2 egg whites

COOKED 2 cups cooked rice

1½ teaspoons grated parmesan

Heat oven to 375 degrees. Liberally coat six cups of a muffin tin with olive oil or nonstick cooking spray.

In a medium bowl, whisk the eggs until they become light and fluffy.

Fold in the cooked rice and mix well. Fill each tin ¾ full and top with a sprinkle of parmesan. Bake for 15 minutes, or until the soufflés are set and the cheese is golden brown.

Let cool to the touch before wrapping. Store in the refrigerator.

TIP Making portables is easier and more efficient when you have your favorite ingredients cooked and ready to go. If you don't have cooked rice on hand, see Appendix C for conversions of cooked ingredients (page 259).

PER SERVING› Energy 138 cal, **Fat** 6 g, **Sodium** 335 mg, **Carbs** 7 g, **Fiber** 0 g, **Protein** 12 g, **Water** 60%

MUSHROOM & SWISS FRITTATA

2 cups sliced mushrooms

½ cup diced onion

¼ cup coarsely chopped parsley

COOKED 2 cups cooked rice

4 eggs, lightly beaten

½ cup shredded Swiss cheese

1 teaspoon celery salt

1 tablespoon grated parmesan

dash of salt and pepper

Heat oven to 350 degrees.

In a nonstick sauté pan, heat a small amount of olive oil to coat bottom evenly. Over medium-high heat, sauté the mushrooms, onion, and parsley until the mushrooms are tender and onions are translucent. Remove from heat and drain any excess oil.

Combine the remaining ingredients in a medium bowl. Stir in the mushroom and onion mixture.

Lightly grease a muffin tin and fill six of the forms ¾ full. Bake 15 minutes or until centers are firm.

Let cool to the touch before wrapping. Store extras in the refrigerator.

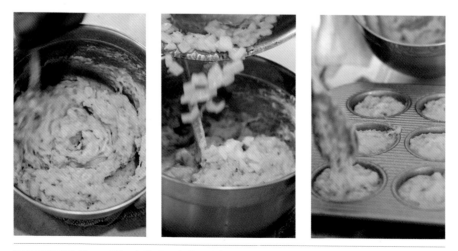

PER SERVING› **Energy** 174 cal, **Fat** 9 g, **Sodium** 292 mg, **Carbs** 15 g, **Fiber** 1 g, **Protein** 9 g, **Water** 65%

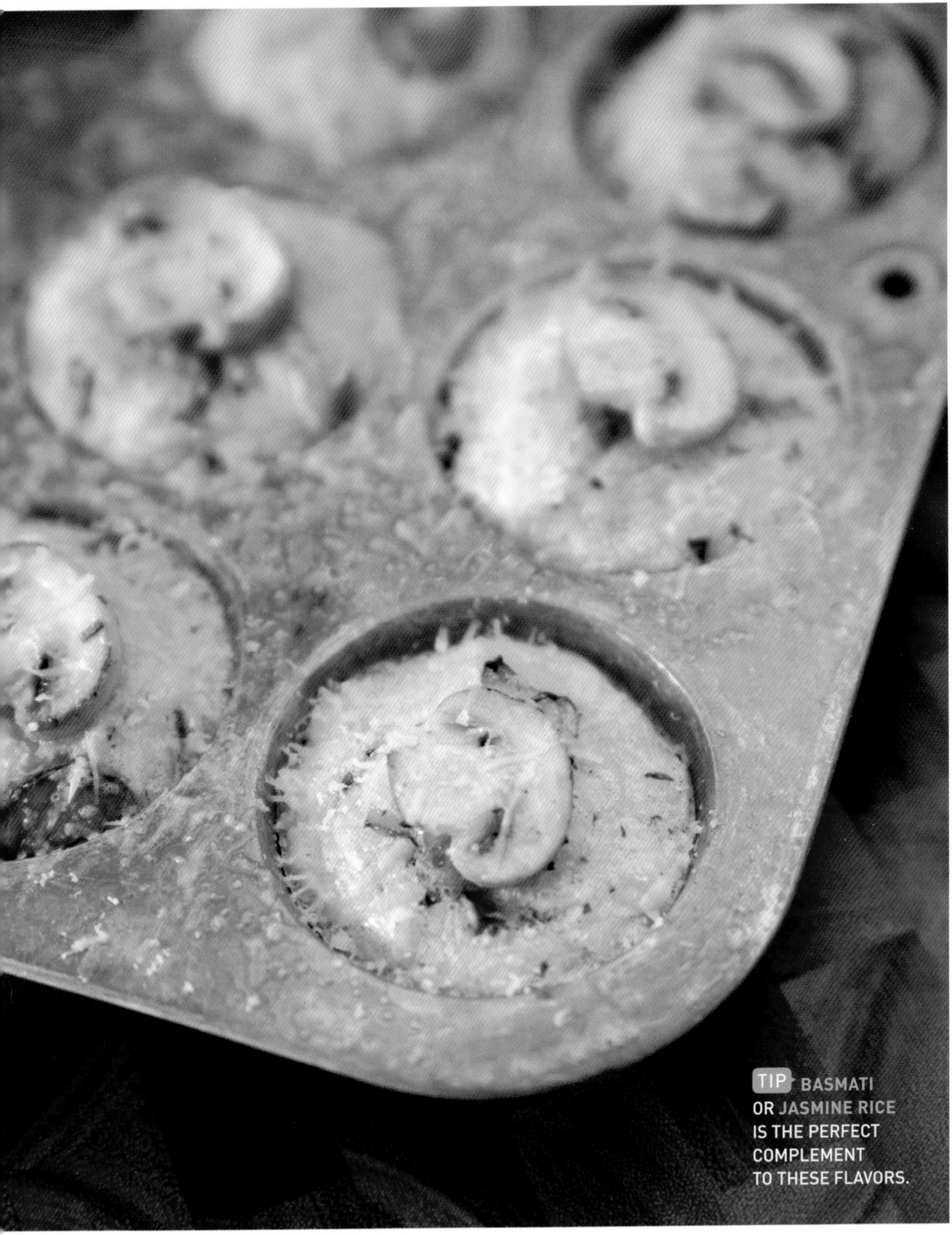

TIP BASMATI
OR JASMINE RICE
IS THE PERFECT
COMPLEMENT
TO THESE FLAVORS.

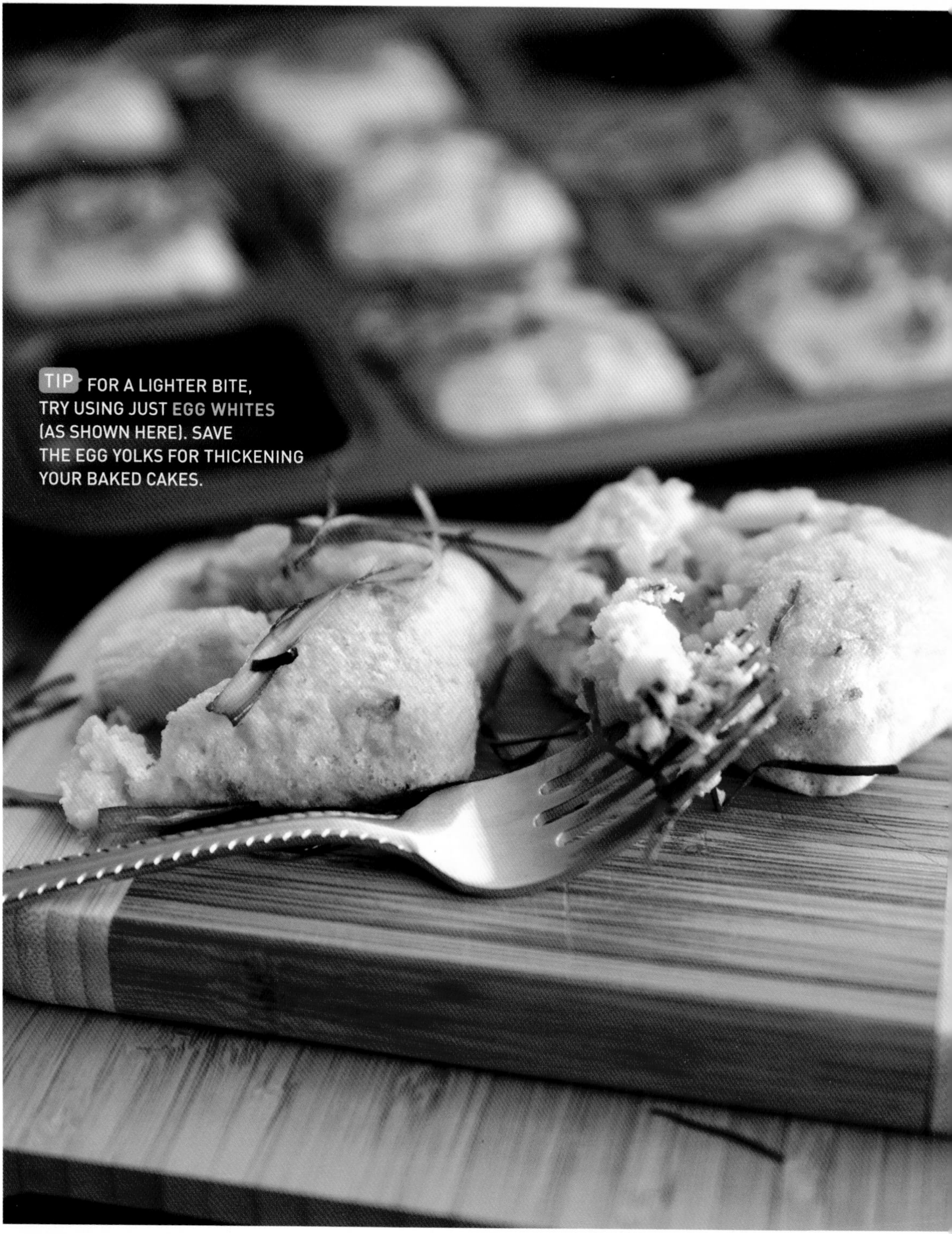

TIP FOR A LIGHTER BITE, TRY USING JUST EGG WHITES (AS SHOWN HERE). SAVE THE EGG YOLKS FOR THICKENING YOUR BAKED CAKES.

POTATO & LEEK FRITTATA

1 medium potato,
peeled and cubed

¼ cup thinly sliced leeks
or green onions

6 egg whites, lightly beaten
(or 4 eggs)

½ cup shredded sharp
cheddar cheese

1 teaspoon Old Bay Seasoning

dash of salt and pepper

4 ounces bacon, chopped
(optional)

Heat oven to 350 degrees.

Place the cubed potatoes in a microwave-safe bowl with a splash of water and cover with plastic wrap. Cook on high until fork-tender, about 3 to 5 minutes. (Or, boil on the stovetop until tender, then drain thoroughly.)

Heat just enough oil to coat a nonstick sauté pan over medium-high heat. Add the leeks and potato. Cook until leeks are bright green and tender.

Combine the remaining ingredients in a medium bowl. Fold in potato and leeks, crushing the potato as you incorporate the ingredients. *Add bacon here if using.*

Lightly grease a muffin tin and fill cups ¾ full. Bake 15 minutes or until centers are firm.

Let cool to the touch before wrapping. Store extras in the refrigerator.

PER SERVING
(6 egg whites)› **Energy** 40 cal, **Fat** 2 g, **Sodium** 111 mg, **Carbs** 3 g, **Fiber** 0 g, **Protein** 3 g, **Water** 65%
(with 4 eggs)› **Energy** 56 cal, **Fat** 3 g, **Sodium** 107 mg, **Carbs** 3 g, **Fiber** 0 g, **Protein** 4 g, **Water** 60%

SPINACH & ZUCCHINI FRITTATA

2 cups zucchini sliced into little "matchsticks"

1 cup packed fresh spinach leaves, chopped small

4 eggs, lightly beaten

2 cups cubed day-old bread, tightly packed

1 tablespoon grated parmesan

1 teaspoon garlic salt

dash of salt and pepper

Heat oven to 350 degrees.

In a nonstick sauté pan, heat enough olive oil to coat bottom evenly. Over medium heat, sauté the zucchini and spinach until the zucchini is tender. Remove from heat and drain any excess oil.

In a medium bowl, lightly beat the eggs. Add the bread and remaining ingredients. Fold in zucchini and spinach.

Lightly grease a muffin tin and fill six of the forms ¾ full. Bake 15 minutes or until centers are firm.

Let cool to the touch before wrapping. Store extras in the refrigerator.

PER SERVING› Energy 104 cal, **Fat** 6 g, **Sodium** 137 mg, **Carbs** 6 g, **Fiber** 1 g, **Protein** 6 g, **Water** 67%

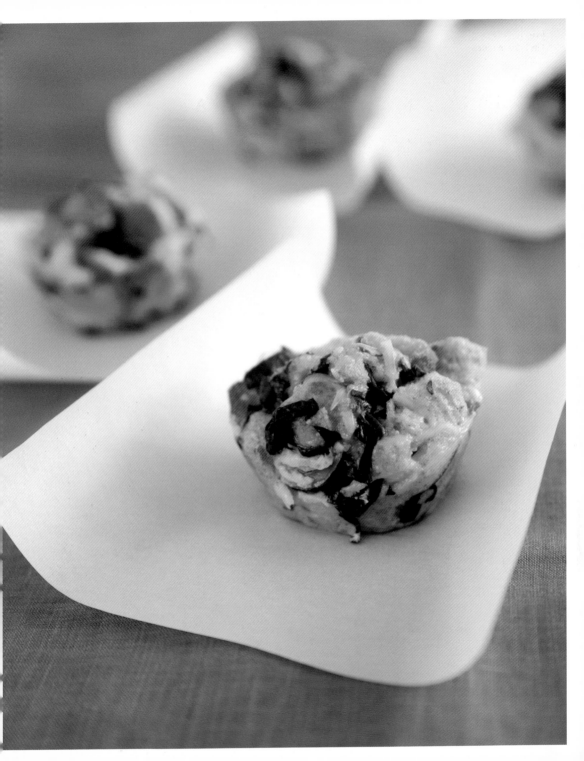

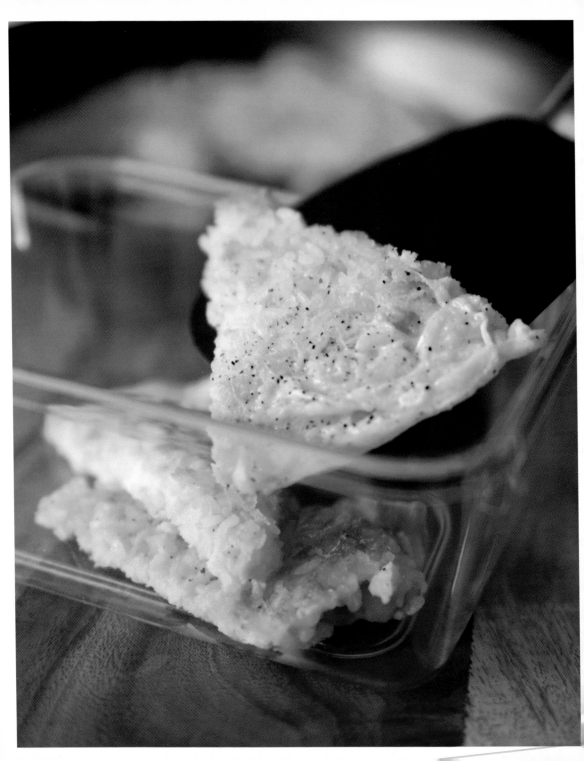

CRISPY RICE OMELET

1 tablespoon olive oil

COOKED   1 cup cooked rice

6 eggs

1½ teaspoons grated parmesan

coarse salt and pepper to taste

Liberally coat a medium nonstick sauté pan with olive oil and place it over high heat.

Once the pan is hot, add the cooked rice to the sauté pan, spread evenly, and cook until crisp (about 3 minutes). Lightly beat the eggs in a medium bowl and pour over the rice. Mix gently, then let the eggs begin to set up.

Loosen the edges of the omelet with a spatula as you tilt the pan, allowing the uncooked eggs to fill in around the edges. Cover and cook until the eggs in the center of the pan set up, or finish in the oven at 350 degrees for about 5 minutes. Top with grated parmesan and a hearty shake of coarse salt and pepper.

Cut into 6 triangles. Let cool to the touch before wrapping. Store extras in the refrigerator.

PER SERVING› Energy 133 cal, **Fat** 8 g, **Sodium** 268 mg, **Carbs** 7 g, **Fiber** 0 g, **Protein** 8 g, **Water** 46%

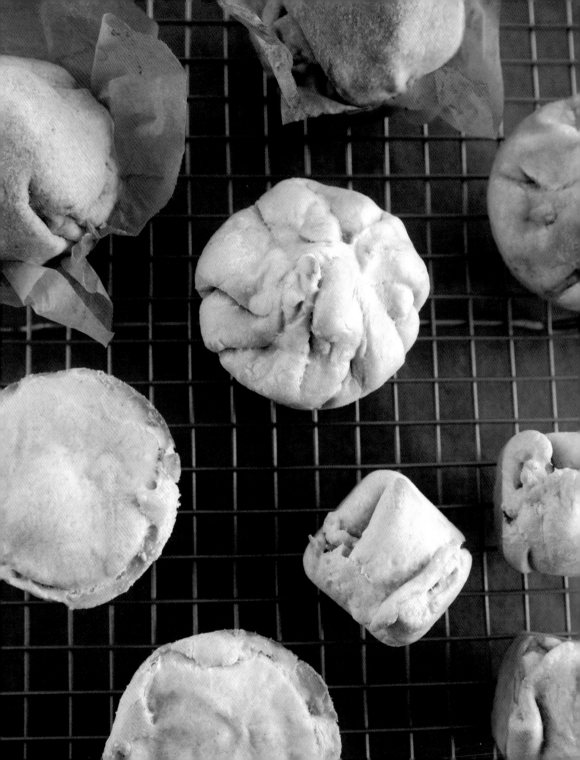

TWO-BITE PIES

Small stuffed pies are the perfect "pocket" for your favorite flavor. While two-bite pies make it look like you've spent hours in the kitchen, with a little practice you can stock up the freezer with a dozen pies in under an hour.

We've included several different crusts, ranging from traditional to gluten-free to our innovative quick crust and warm dough versions. If it's a burrito you're craving, any of the savory pie fillings can be piled into a tortilla for a bigger bite.

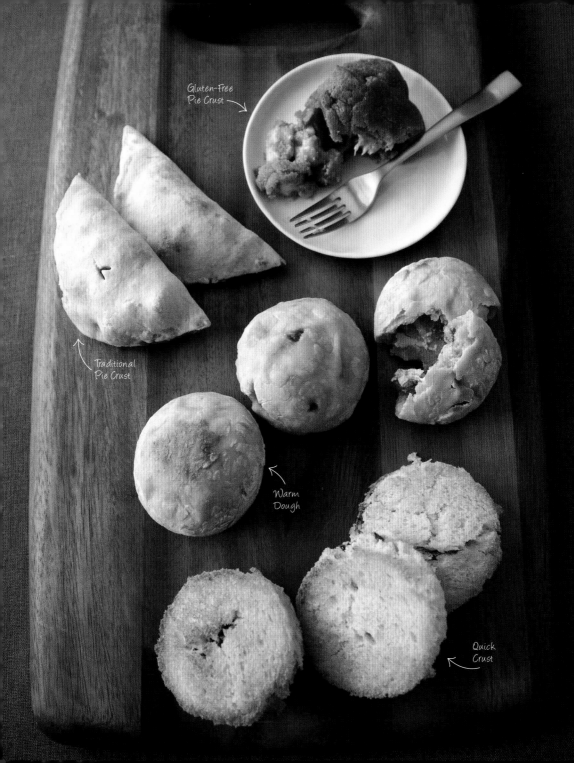

Gluten-Free
Pie Crust

Traditional
Pie Crust

Warm
Dough

Quick
Crust

V VEGETARIAN   G GLUTEN-FREE

PROCESS

☆ Choose your pie crust.

☆ Mix up a sweet or savory filling.

☆ Decide how to prep and present your pies: muffin tin or turnover, simple or high-class.

☆ Jam the filling inside and bake in the oven.

TIME› 15 minutes hands-on,
30–60 minutes to chill

TRADITIONAL PIE CRUST

Traditional pie crusts work well with any filling and can be kept frozen for weeks.

3 cups flour

½ teaspoon salt

½ teaspoon ground cinnamon (optional)

⅔ cup cold unsalted butter, cut into ½-inch cubes

½ cup cold water

In a small food processor pulse together flour, salt, and cinnamon. Add butter and blend until the butter pieces are no longer visible.

Transfer the mixture to a large bowl and add cold water a little bit at a time, using a spatula to turn the dough and mix ingredients. Add more water or a bit more flour until the dough begins to take shape. Divide dough into 12 portions and pat each one into a firm ball.

Wrap and chill the dough before handling (at least 30 minutes in the freezer or 1 hour in the refrigerator).

You might have leftover dough if you are making sweet pies.

PER SERVING
(12 servings)› **Energy** 204 cal, **Fat** 10 g, **Sodium** 99 mg, **Carbs** 24 g, **Fiber** 1 g, **Protein** 3 g, **Water** 18%

TURNOVER PIE PREP ✚ BEST WITH TRADITIONAL PIE CRUST

Heat oven to 350 degrees. Prepare a baking sheet with nonstick cooking spray or parchment paper.

On a lightly floured surface, roll out or press out each ball of dough to be approximately 6 inches round, about ⅛-inch thick. Place a generous scoop of the pie filling on one-half of the dough.

Lightly brush the edge of the crust with water. Fold dough over the filling and press the edges together with your fingertips. Use a dull knife and trim up the edges, creating a seal.

Place pies on a baking sheet and bake for 15 minutes.

Let the pies rest 10 minutes before removing them from the baking sheet. Cool completely before wrapping.

TIP Brush the top of the crust with coconut oil, butter, or egg wash before you place them in the oven. **EGG WASH** = 1 egg white + 1½ teaspoons cold water whisked together

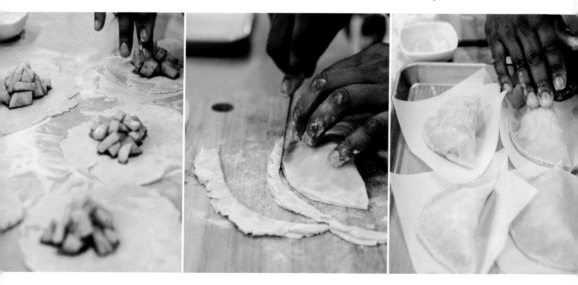

GLUTEN-FREE PIE CRUST

Most gluten-free recipes are loaded with special flours and obscure ingredients. The ingenuity of this pie crust is that we just use about half a loaf of gluten-free bread from the freezer. There's a wide variety available at your local grocery store. A soft, moist bread will bind well with a modest amount of butter or coconut oil.

4 cups cubed gluten-free bread, tightly packed (~20 ounces)

2 tablespoons butter, cut into cubes

1 egg, lightly beaten

1½ teaspoons apple juice or cold water (optional)

Softened coconut oil can be used in place of butter, depending on the flavor you want to create.

Place the gluten-free bread in a food processor and pulse until it breaks down into a fine mixture.

Add butter and pulse until it is incorporated. Mix in the egg. If the dough seems too dry, add juice or water in small increments, just enough to hold the crust together. The dough will be a little soft.

Divide dough into 12 equal parts and shape each one into a firm ball, a bit larger than a golf ball.

Wrap and chill the dough in the refrigerator for at least 1 hour before rolling it out. If you place this dough in the freezer, allow at least 30 minutes to thaw. Gluten-free dough will need to be worked—just be patient with it.

You might have leftover dough if you are making sweet pies.

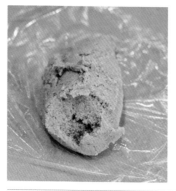

GLUTEN-FREE DOUGH will be a bit softer than traditional pie crust. It bakes up light and moist, which makes it ideal for eating on a ride.

PER SERVING
(12 servings)› **Energy** 159 cal, **Fat** 6 g, **Sodium** 292 mg, **Carbs** 21 g, **Fiber** 1 g, **Protein** 4 g, **Water** 12%

MUFFIN-TIN PIE PREP ⊕ USE WITH ANY PIE CRUST

Heat oven to 350 degrees. Generously coat a muffin tin with nonstick cooking spray.

On a lightly floured surface, roll or press out each ball of dough to be large enough to fit into the form and fold back over the filling. *To roll out a gluten-free crust, place each ball of dough between two sheets of plastic and work it slowly.*

Transfer the dough into the muffin forms, gently pressing into place and letting excess dough hang over the edges. Add pie filling level with the top of the muffin tin.

Fold the excess dough over the filling. Add a small disc of dough to fill any gaps, especially if your filling is less dense. Gently press the dough together to create a seal. (If your pies hold together well, turn them upside down in the muffin cups.)

Bake for 15 minutes or until the crust turns golden. Gluten-free crust will not completely change color, but it will take on a slightly richer color as it cooks.

When you remove the pies from the oven, run a plastic knife around the perimeter of each pie. Let the pies rest 10 minutes before removing them from the pan. Cool completely before wrapping.

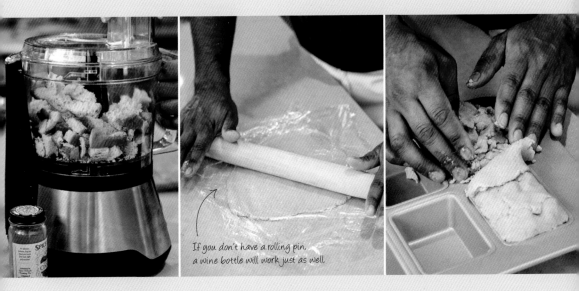

If you don't have a rolling pin, a wine bottle will work just as well

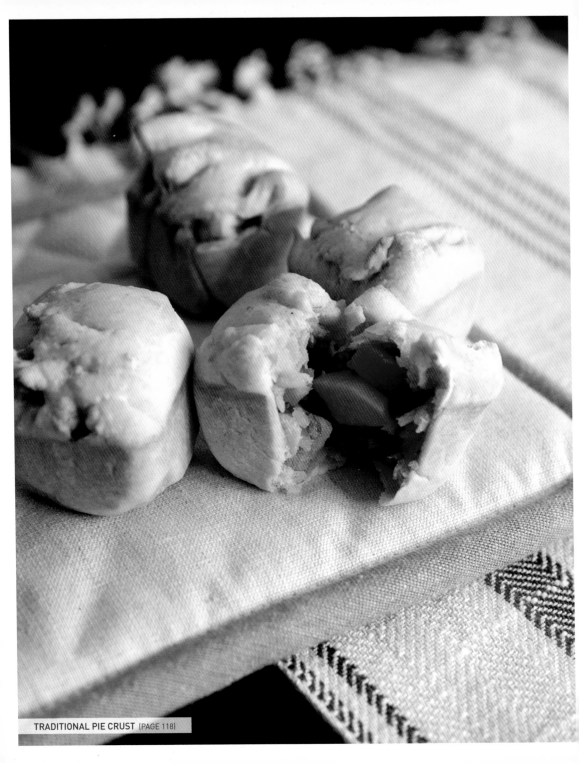

TRADITIONAL PIE CRUST [PAGE 118]

BEEF & SWEET POTATO PIES

8 ounces grass-fed ground beef

1 medium sweet potato, peeled and cubed (~1 cup)

1 tablespoon liquid aminos or low-sodium soy sauce

1 tablespoon brown sugar

1 tablespoon red wine vinegar

1 teaspoon coarse sea salt

1 teaspoon ground cinnamon

COOKED 2 cups cooked rice

In a nonstick sauté pan over medium-high heat, cook the ground beef until browned. Drain excess grease.

Cook the cubed sweet potato in the microwave until fork-tender, about 3 to 5 minutes.

Combine the cooked ground beef and sweet potato in a bowl. Using a wooden spoon, crush the potato as you season the mixture with the soy sauce, brown sugar, red wine vinegar, sea salt, and cinnamon.

Fold in the rice.

Set aside the filling to cool as you prep the dough.

PER SERVING
(Filling)› **Energy** 79 cal, **Fat** 2 g, **Sodium** 375 mg, **Carbs** 10 g, **Fiber** 1 g, **Protein** 4 g, **Water** 61%

SERVINGS› 12
TIME› 20 minutes hands-on,
10–20 minutes in oven

CURRY POTATO & CHICKEN PIES

2 medium potatoes,
peeled and cubed

¼ cup diced onion

½ cup ground chicken

2 teaspoons curry powder

¼ cup golden raisins

¾ cup water

1 tablespoon potato flour

1 tablespoon minced
fresh cilantro

1 teaspoon coarse salt

*You can use minced cooked chicken in
place of the ground chicken. Just add it
to the mixture along with the curry
powder and other ingredients.*

Place the cubed potatoes in a microwave-safe bowl with a splash of water and cover with plastic wrap. Cook on high in the microwave until fork-tender, about 3 to 5 minutes. (Or, boil on the stovetop until tender, then drain thoroughly.)

Coat a sauté pan with oil and bring to medium-high heat. Sauté the onions until translucent, then add the ground chicken and sauté until it is crisp and browned. Drain any excess fat.

Stir in the cooked potatoes and continue to cook until the potatoes become golden brown.

Add the remaining ingredients and cook until most of the water evaporates, mashing the potatoes as you stir.

Set aside filling to cool as you prep the dough.

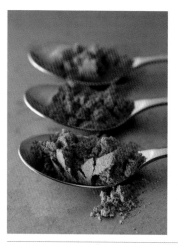

No two **CURRIES** are the same,
so be sure to taste and adjust
the seasoning as needed.

PER SERVING
(Filling)› **Energy** 52 cal, **Fat** 2 g, **Sodium** 160 mg, **Carbs** 7 g, **Fiber** 1 g, **Protein** 2 g, **Water** 65%

TIP SAVORY PIES MAKE
A FANTASTIC APPETIZER FOR
YOUR NEXT DINNER PARTY.
LINE EACH MUFFIN FORM WITH
A SQUARE OF PARCHMENT PAPER.

TRADITIONAL PIE CRUST [PAGE 118]

★ ★ ★

"Recipes from *Feed Zone* are my new, not-so-secret training tool. They deliver huge taste and even bigger performance benefits. My third consecutive women's course record at the Leadville Trail 100 is proof."

REBECCA RUSCH
4-TIME WINNER LEADVILLE TRAIL 100
3-TIME 24-HOUR SOLO MOUNTAIN BIKE
WORLD CHAMPION

Regardless of your athletic talent or aspirations, the foods that fuel you are best when made, as much as possible, from scratch and with *real intent & care*.

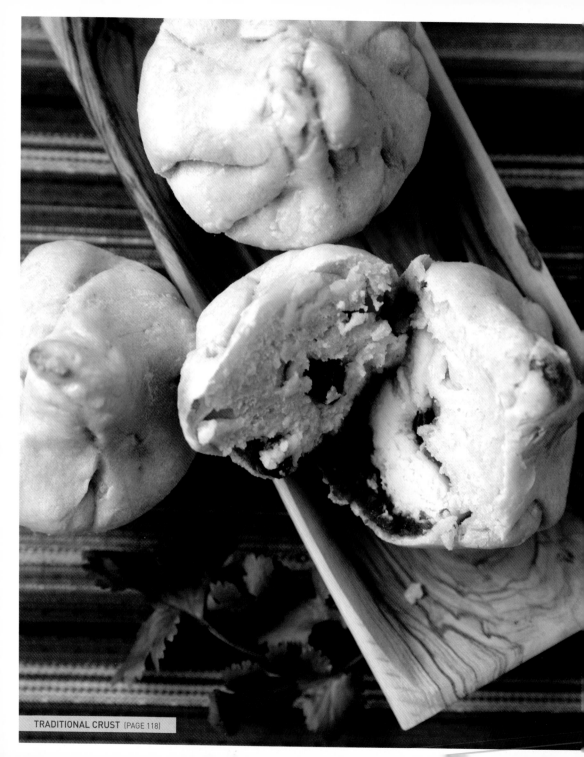

TRADITIONAL CRUST [PAGE 118]

BLACK BEAN & PEANUT MOLÉ PIES

**1 cup canned black beans,
rinsed and drained**

½ cup chopped carrot

Bring a lightly oiled sauté pan to medium-high heat. Add the black beans and carrot and cook until the carrots soften. Remove from heat.

For a spicier pie, mix in molé here.

1 cup soy milk, heated

1½ cups potato flakes

1 teaspoon coarse salt

Heat the soy milk in the microwave for 90 seconds. In a mixing bowl, combine potato flakes with hot milk and stir vigorously to incorporate.

**1 cup Molé Sauce
(recipe on page 130)**

Set aside fillings to cool as you prep the dough.

TIP To keep the flavor relatively mild, build your pies using a dollop of the molé sauce and a heaping spoonful of the potato mixture. Top with a spoonful of the bean and carrot mixture.

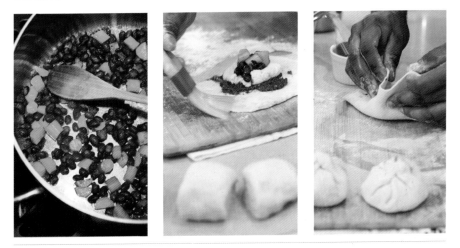

PER SERVING
(Filling & Sauce)› **Energy** 105 cal, **Fat** 5 g, **Sodium** 219 mg, **Carbs** 13 g, **Fiber** 3 g, **Protein** 4 g, **Water** 18%

MOLÉ SAUCE

1 cup raw shelled peanuts, crushed

2 tablespoons tomato paste

¼ cup raisins

½ cup semisweet chocolate chips

1 cup water

1½ teaspoons ground cinnamon

1½ teaspoons ancho chili powder

Ancho chili powder has a smoky taste that complements the flavors of molé, but any chili powder will do.

In a dry saucepan over medium-high heat, combine the peanuts and raisins. Stir briskly as the nuts begin to toast and the raisins plump, about 5 minutes.

Reduce heat to low, add the tomato paste, then mix in chocolate chips and stir until they melt. Finish by adding water. Simmer on low for 5 minutes.

Mix in the remaining ingredients and adjust flavor with salt, if needed.

Transfer the mixture to a blender or small food processor and pulse until the nuts and raisins are incorporated. The finished sauce will not be completely smooth. Don't overprocess—too much air will change the color. You want a rich, chocolate brown color with hits of toasted red.

Makes about 2½ cups of molé sauce. Store leftover sauce in an airtight container in the refrigerator for up to 10 days. Use it to top off burritos, chicken, or beef.

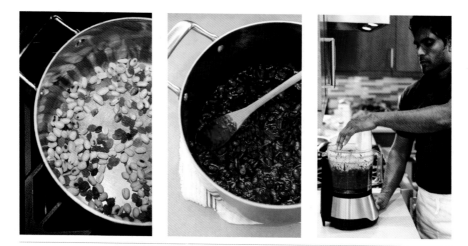

Nutrition facts for full recipe can be found in Appendix A.

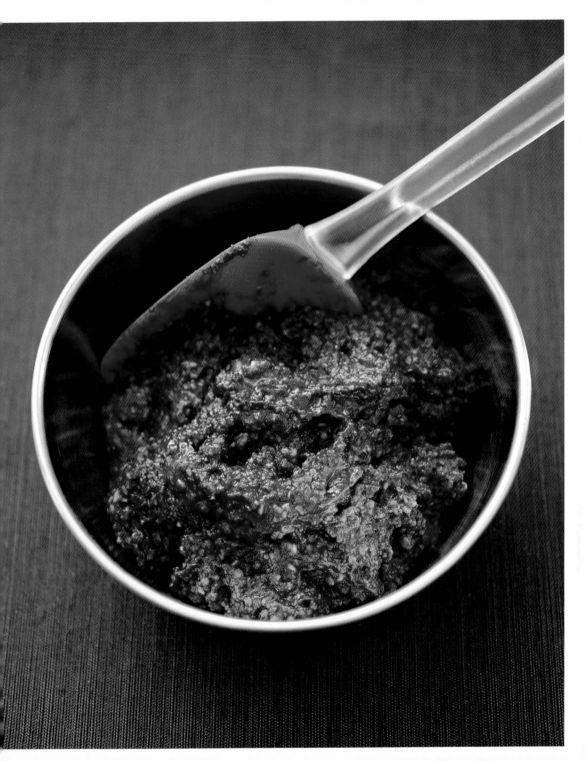

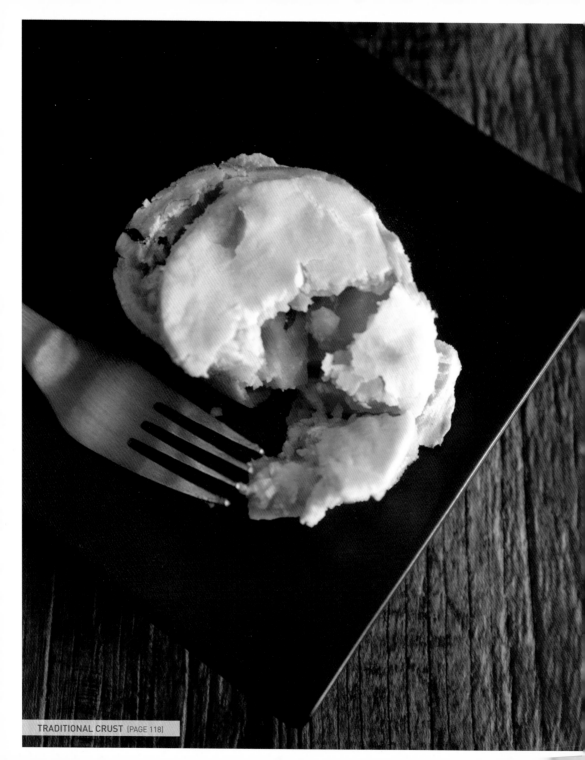

TRADITIONAL CRUST [PAGE 118]

GOLDEN BEET & CHICKEN POT PIE

½ cup golden beets, peeled and cubed

8 ounces ground chicken or minced chicken breast

½ cup chopped carrots

2 tablespoons diced celery

1 tablespoon minced onion

1 vegetable bouillon cube

½ cup potato flakes

¾ cup water

If you can't find golden beets, use any other variety.

Steam or microwave the beets for 10 minutes or until they are soft.

While the beets are steaming, bring a lightly oiled sauté pan to medium-high heat and cook the chicken until it begins to show a hint of brown.

Add the carrots, celery, and onion, stirring periodically until the carrots soften and the onions become translucent.

Stir in the steamed beets, bouillon cube, potato flakes, and water. Once the bouillon is fully incorporated in the mixture and the water is absorbed, add salt to taste.

Set aside filling to cool slightly as you prep the dough.

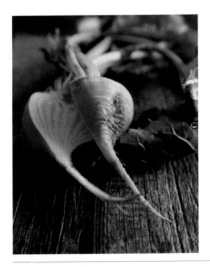

BEETS are most commonly deep red-purple in color, but come in a wide variety of other shades, including golden yellow and red-and-white striped.

PER SERVING
(Filling) › Energy 52 cal, **Fat** 3 g, **Sodium** 442 mg, **Carbs** 3 g, **Fiber** 1 g, **Protein** 4 g, **Water** 67%

FAST-TRACK YOUR PIES

Both the traditional and gluten-free crusts require some extra time to chill the dough. Our warm dough lets you skip that step, and the quick crust simply uses slices of a loaf of soft bread as crust. For the times when you need food fast, just wrap up any savory pie filling in a tortilla and you'll have 6 delicious burritos ready in no time.

WARM DOUGH

This dough can be worked with your hands while it is still warm, saving you valuable time. Made without butter or oil, warm dough is slightly dense, but the resulting pies are easy to eat and incredibly portable.

3 cups flour

1 teaspoon sugar

2 cups almond milk, heated

Heat the oven to 350 degrees. Lightly grease a baking sheet or line with parchment paper.

Combine the flour and sugar in a medium bowl and stir to combine.

Heat the milk in the microwave for 2 minutes on high. While it is still hot, pour the milk into the flour mixture and stir well with a wooden spoon. As the dough begins to cool slightly and hold together, work it with your hands, dividing into 12 portions, each slightly larger than a golf ball.

Flatten each ball of dough in your hand (it will be thicker than the other doughs) and add a spoonful of filling. Pull and pinch the dough over the top of the filling.

Place the stuffed pies upside down on the baking sheet and brush tops with butter or oil. Bake for 10–15 minutes or until the pies are slightly brown on top.

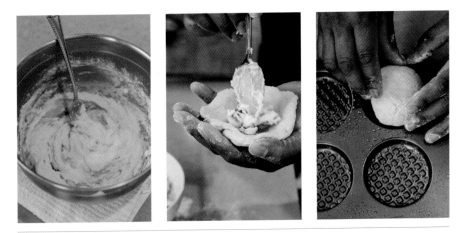

PER SERVING
(12 servings)› **Energy** 124 cal, **Fat** 1 g, **Sodium** 24 mg, **Carbs** 25 g, **Fiber** 1 g, **Protein** 3 g, **Water** 19%

HOW TO MAKE A QUICK CRUST

For this crust, simply pull out a loaf of your favorite soft bread. Potato and buttermilk are easy varieties to work with. Soft wheat breads work too, though they have more fiber.

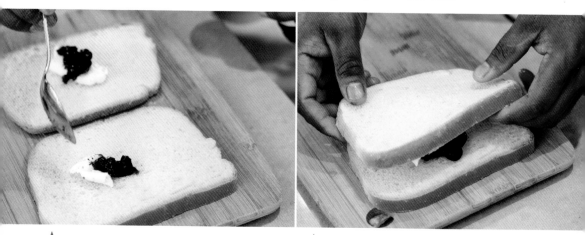

⭐1 Start with two slices of soft bread. Add a heaping spoonful of filling and brush a bit of water around it. (This will help seal the edge.)

⭐2 Top with another slice of bread.

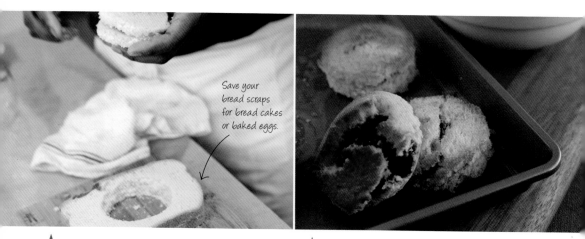

Save your bread scraps for bread cakes or baked eggs.

⭐5 Brush the pies with melted butter or olive oil and place on a baking sheet.

⭐6 Bake at 350 degrees for 15 minutes, or until the bread is toasted.

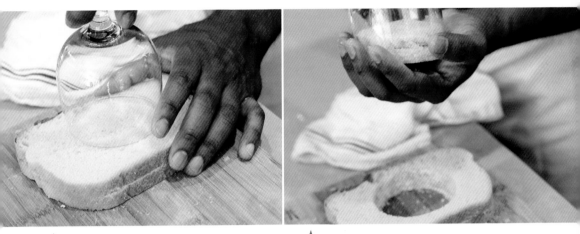

⭐ Use a dull-rimmed glass to press the two "crusts" together.

⭐ If the pie sticks inside the glass, use a butter knife to gently pop it out.

TO USE A QUICK CRUST IN A MUFFIN TIN

Roll out the bread slices using a rolling pin or wine bottle. Cut off bread crust.

Brush a bit of butter or olive oil into each muffin tin. (This will help keep the bread moist.)

Press the bread into each muffin form.

Add filling.

Make a top crust by taking the excess bread and folding it over the center. Or, lay a small piece of pressed bread over the top of the pie. Wet the edges of the bread and pinch together.

Brush the top of the pie with melted butter or olive oil. Bake at 350 degrees for 15 minutes, or until bread is toasted.

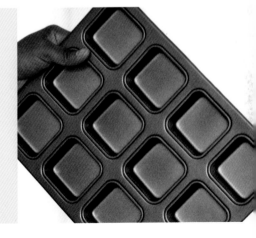

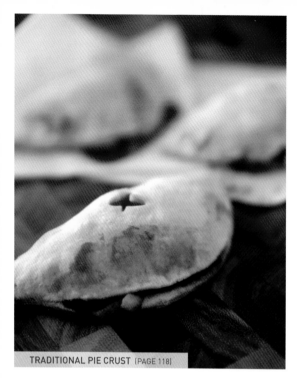

TRADITIONAL PIE CRUST [PAGE 118]

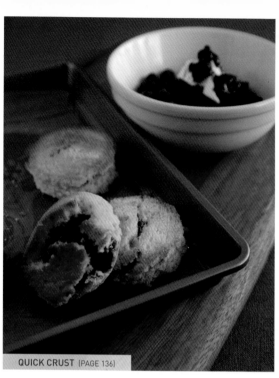

QUICK CRUST [PAGE 136]

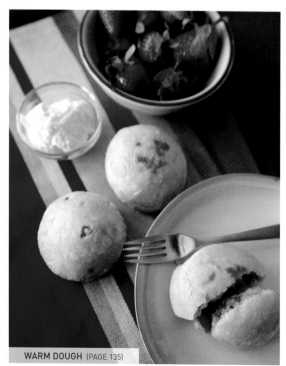

WARM DOUGH [PAGE 135]

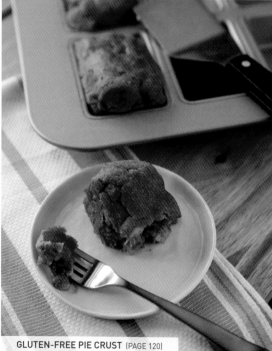

GLUTEN-FREE PIE CRUST [PAGE 120]

SWEET TWO-BITE PIES

Fruit pies work well with any crust and they double as a tasty dessert. If you plan to enjoy them on a ride, use just 1–2 tablespoons of filling in each pie to limit fiber. Let the pies cool completely after baking so the filling firms up.

APPLE

2 cups diced apples (peeled)

½ cup brown sugar

2 teaspoons ground cinnamon or pumpkin pie spice

1 teaspoon vanilla extract

1 teaspoon coarse salt

Choose a firm apple like Granny Smith or Honeycrisp for best results. In the summer, substitute fresh peaches.

BLUEBERRY

1 cup fresh blueberries

½ cup blueberry preserves

¼ cup cream cheese

sprinkle brown sugar to taste

STRAWBERRIES & CREAM

2 cups fresh strawberries, sliced lengthwise

2 tablespoons strawberry preserves

¼ cup ricotta or cottage cheese

BANANA WALNUT

2 large bananas, diced ← *Firm bananas work best.*

¼ cup finely chopped walnuts

1 tablespoon brown sugar

1 teaspoon ground cinnamon or your favorite baking spice

TO MAKE FRUIT PIE FILLING

Mix all ingredients together in a bowl and **PAIR** with the pie crust of your choice. Use just enough dough to wrap the fruit mixture, trimming off the excess.

If you use a traditional or gluten-free crust, you might find you have some dough left over.

Nutrition facts for Sweet Two-Bite Pie fillings can be found in Appendix A.

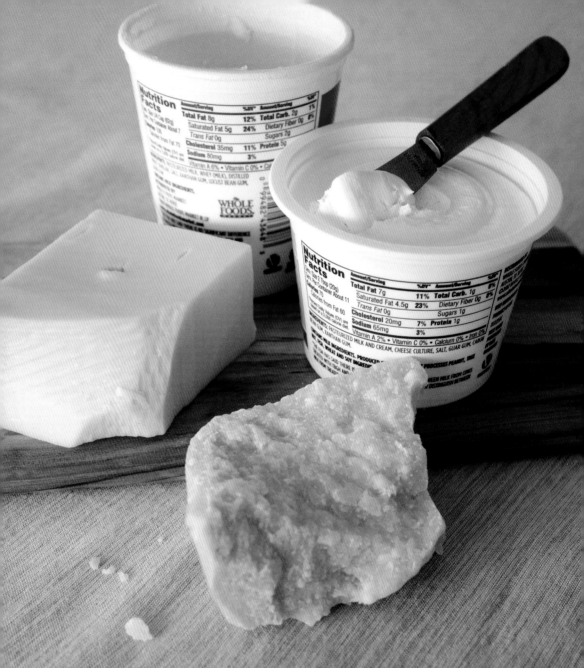

CHEESE AND CREAM CHEESE are very common in the European peloton. Small sandwiches with cheese, jam, and prosciutto are considered classics (see page 243). Less than a teaspoon of ricotta or cream cheese per pie gives a huge flavor boost. If you have trouble with dairy, substitute nut butter or just leave it out.

What you call your diet or how you label it is far less important than the ingredients you use to build it. ⋆ Like proper training, *the inherent quality and diversity of what we choose to eat* is key to optimal health and performance.

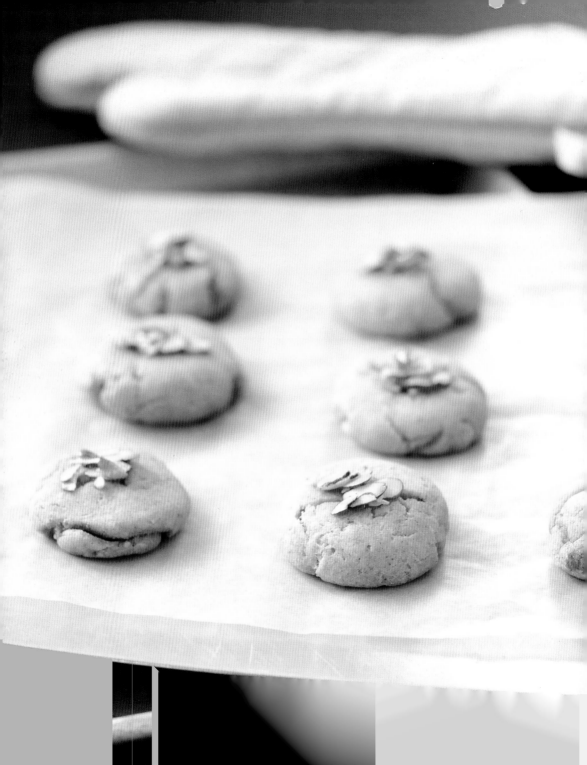

BAKED CAKES & COOKIES

Every athlete should eat more cupcakes. Well, these aren't exactly your average cupcake. Our baked cakes are not overly sweet, but they are every bit as indulgent as a cupcake when you are on the go. And if you need another hit of sugar, no one has to know.

Featuring plenty of eggs and a variety of carbs, these cakes and cookies work for endurance athletes because they are nutrient dense without being dry. Meaning they stand up to Allen's couch potato test—you could enjoy them whether you are on the bike or on the couch (though you'll definitely want to hold off on the extra sugar on the days you are just sitting on the couch).

V VEGETARIAN   **G** GLUTEN-FREE

CHANGE IT UP› BAKED CAKES MANY WAYS

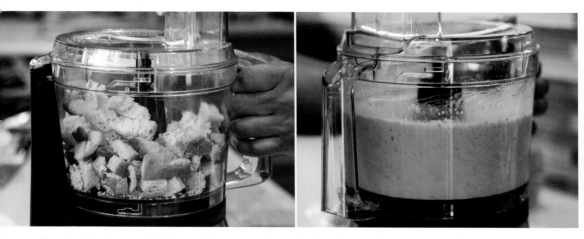

Our bread cakes are delicious, whether you leave the bread cubes intact or puree them into the batter.

CHUNKY BATTER = rich, bread-pudding texture
PUREED BATTER = lighter, cake-like texture

We briefly pulsed the chocolate cakes to have the best of both worlds.

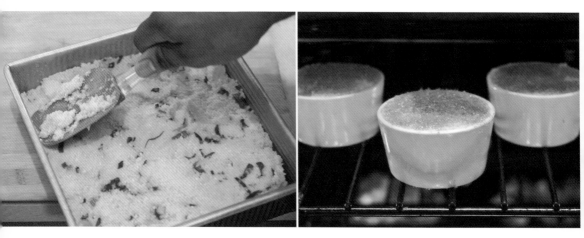

Corn cakes will cook on the stovetop and set in the pan as they cool. But you can finish them any way you like.

COOL & CUT = moist, soft texture
PAN FRY OR BROIL = crispy edges

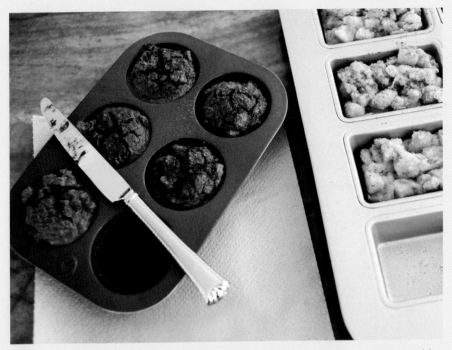

BAKED CAKES work in a variety of different pans. Decide how big you want your bite to be and use the guidelines below to adjust baking times and servings. Or keep it simple—all of these recipes work in a standard muffin tin.

PAN	BAKING TIME	NOTES
8" or 9" square baking pan	35–40 minutes	Let cool before cutting into 12 squares.
9" × 5" loaf pan	25–30 minutes	Let cool before cutting into 6 thick slices. Half a slice is the perfect portable.
Muffin pan	15–20 minutes	12 easy individual servings
Mini muffin pan	8–10 minutes	Makes 24 mini muffins, 2 per serving. Use a spread and stack them.

Baking times will vary from one oven to the next. The center of the cake should be set firm—a toothpick inserted in the center of the cake will come out clean. Also note that baking time will change the moisture content. Nutrition facts include moisture content after baking in a standard muffin tin for 15–20 minutes.

SERVINGS› 12
TIME› 10 minutes prep,
20–25 minutes in the oven

SAUSAGE & POTATO CAKES

3 large potatoes,
peeled and cubed

4 ounces chicken sausage

¼ cup minced onion

4 eggs

½ cup flour

1 teaspoon salt

1 teaspoon ground cumin

1 tablespoon grated parmesan

OPTIONAL ADDITIONS

1 tablespoon chopped
fresh basil or parsley

Heat oven to 350 degrees. Lightly coat a muffin tin with nonstick cooking spray.

Place the potatoes in a microwave-safe bowl with a splash of water and cover with plastic wrap. Cook on high in the microwave for 3–5 minutes. (Or, boil on stovetop until tender. Drain thoroughly.)

In a dry nonstick sauté pan over medium heat, brown the sausage, then add potatoes and onions, cooking until potato edges begin to crisp. Set aside and let cool.

Mix together eggs, flour, salt, and cumin. Beat the mixture until the eggs become light, then add to the potato mixture.

Add basil or parsley here if using.

Press mixture into muffin tin, sprinkle tops with parmesan and additional chicken sausage if you like, and bake 20–25 minutes or until a toothpick inserted into the center comes out clean.

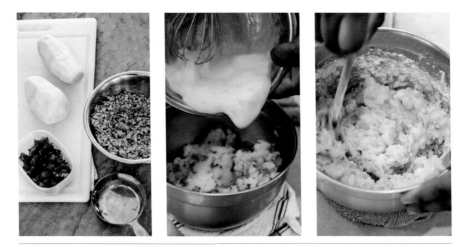

PER SERVING› Energy 107 cal, **Fat** 4 g, **Sodium** 402 mg, **Carbs** 13 g, **Fiber** 1 g, **Protein** 5 g, **Water** 53%
Nutrition facts for optional additions can be found in Appendix B.

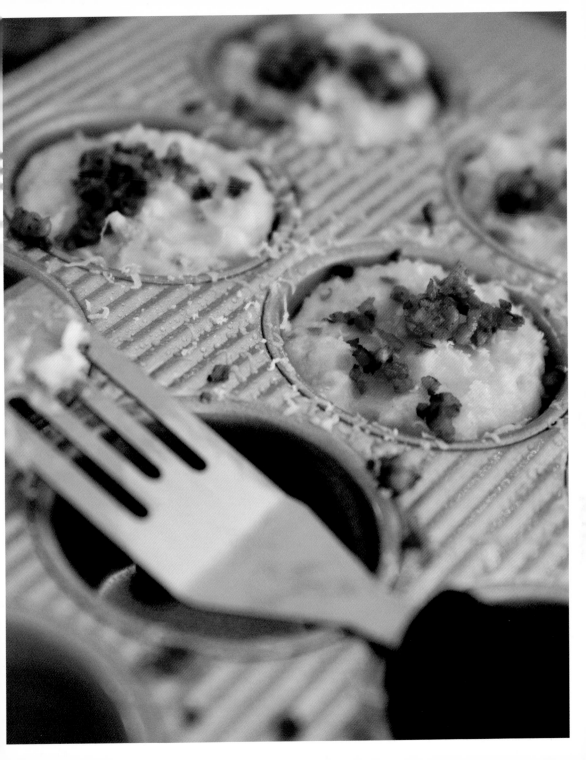

TIP FOR A DIFFERENT FINISH, PAN-FRY OR BROIL THE INDIVIDUAL CAKES UNTIL THEIR EDGES BECOME CRISP.

SPINACH & RED PEPPER POLENTA CAKES

6 cups water

2 cups uncooked polenta

2 cubes vegetable bouillon (optional)

2 tablespoons minced red bell pepper

1 cup shredded spinach, loosely packed

¼ cup crumbled feta (or any crumbly cheese)

2 teaspoons raw sugar

1 teaspoon coarse salt

Lightly coat an 8" square baking pan with nonstick cooking spray.

On the stovetop, bring water with a dash of salt to a boil and slowly stir in polenta. Reduce heat and simmer, stirring frequently to prevent sticking. Cook for 20–30 minutes.

If using bouillon, add here in place of salt.

Stir in the peppers. Cook for 5–10 minutes longer, or until mixture thickens.

Remove from heat. Stir in the spinach and cheese and adjust flavor to taste.

Pour mixture into pan and let set for 10–15 minutes to firm up. Mix the raw sugar and coarse salt in a small bowl and sprinkle on top.

Cut into squares.

BOUILLON CUBES bring more flavor to rice, polenta, or grits. Look for a high-quality organic brand without extra additives.

PER SERVING› Energy 112 cal, Fat 1 g, Sodium 289 mg, Carbs 22 g, Fiber 1 g, Protein 3 g, Water 71%

CRISPY GRITS

4 cups water

2 cups uncooked grits

COOKED ½ cup cooked
crumbled bacon

2 tablespoons fresh thyme
(or any fresh herbs you
have on hand)

¼ cup grated parmesan

2 teaspoons raw sugar

1 teaspoon coarse salt

1½ teaspoons olive oil (to fry)

Lightly coat a muffin tin or an 8" square baking pan
with nonstick cooking spray.

Bring water with a dash of salt to a boil in a
saucepan over high heat. Add grits and stir
frequently for 3–4 minutes. The mixture will begin
to thicken. Remove from heat and stir in cooked
bacon and thyme.

Pour cooked grits into muffin tin or baking pan
and sprinkle with parmesan and a pinch of sugar
and salt. Let set for 10–15 minutes to firm up.

*Cut into squares. Pan-fry the individual squares over
medium-high heat until the edges are golden.*

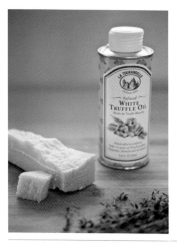

Finishing oils like **TRUFFLE OIL** can
add a wonderful intensity to simple dishes.
Add just a small amount before serving.

PER SERVING› Energy 120 cal, **Fat** 2 g, **Sodium** 188 mg, **Carbs** 21 g, **Fiber** 0 g, **Protein** 3 g, **Water** 64%

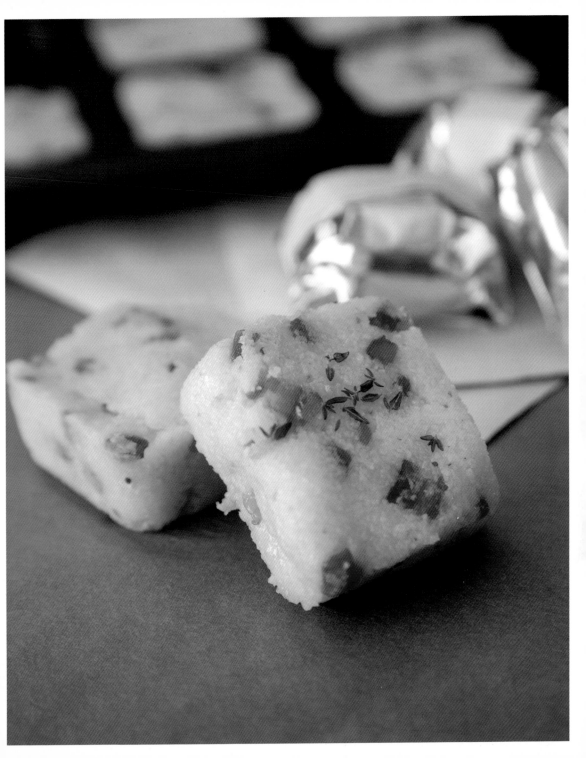

TIP BREAD CAKES ARE FREEZER-FRIENDLY. STORE A PARTIAL LOAF IN A ZIPLOCK BAG AND LET IT THAW OVERNIGHT FOR YOUR NEXT BIG RIDE.

MUSHROOM & THYME BREAD CAKE

8 ounces mushrooms, sliced

¼ cup onion, minced

4 cups cubed gluten-free bread, tightly packed (~half a loaf)

4 eggs, lightly beaten

1 cup soy milk

2 tablespoons fresh thyme leaves

2 teaspoons Old Bay Seasoning (or your favorite seasoning)

1 teaspoon coarse salt

OPTIONAL ADDITIONS

¼ cup grated parmesan

4 ounces chicken sausage

Heat oven to 375 degrees. Lightly coat a standard 9" × 5" loaf pan with nonstick cooking spray.

Bring a dry sauté pan to medium-high heat and add the mushrooms and onion. Once the mushrooms have browned just a bit, remove from heat. *Add chicken sausage here if using.*

Put all ingredients in a large bowl and stir to combine. *Add parmesan here if using, or sprinkle on top after baking.*

Transfer the mixture to the loaf pan, pressing edges to keep the mixture even. Bake until the cake has set firm and a toothpick inserted in center comes out clean, about 25–30 minutes.

Once the cake has cooled, cut into 6 thick slices and wrap. Half of one thick slice makes for a perfect portable.

TIP A square baking pan or a standard muffin tin will also work here. See chart for different cooking times, page 145.

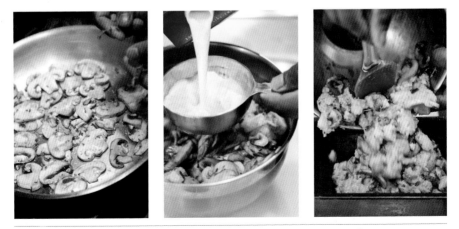

PER SERVING› Energy 99 cal, **Fat** 4 g, **Sodium** 342 mg, **Carbs** 12 g, **Fiber** 1 g, **Protein** 5 g, **Water** 62%
Nutrition facts for optional additions can be found in Appendix B.

A book of recipes won't do much for us unless we **remember to stay active**. ★ This is especially true since *everything that might be good for us when we are exercising or sweating is likely bad for us when we are sitting on our butts*.

★ ★ ★

"Training is a good excuse to inhale more of the goodness coming out of Biju's oven."

GEORGE BENNETT
RADIOSHACK-LEOPARD-TREK PRO CYCLING TEAM
SILVER MEDALIST, NEW ZEALAND NATIONAL
CHAMPIONSHIPS, ROAD RACING

SERVINGS› 12
TIME› 5 minutes prep,
15–35 minutes in oven

FRENCH TOAST CAKES

1 cup almond milk, heated

4 eggs + 1 egg yolk

1 tablespoon raw sugar

1 teaspoon vanilla extract

½ teaspoon ground cinnamon

**4 cups cubed bread,
tightly packed**

Heat oven to 350 degrees. Lightly coat the cups of a muffin tin or an 8" square baking pan with nonstick cooking spray.

Heat the almond milk in the microwave on high for about 90 seconds. Meanwhile, whisk together eggs and egg yolk in a medium bowl.

Add the warm milk, sugar, vanilla, and cinnamon to the eggs. Beat the mixture until the eggs become light.

Fold in bread cubes. Spoon into muffin tin or baking pan, evenly distributing the bread.

Bake muffins for 15–20 minutes and larger cakes for 30 minutes, just until a toothpick inserted into the center comes out clean. If the bread cubes begin to brown and the cakes are not yet fully cooked, cover pan with foil and let bake 5 more minutes.

Top with a sprinkle of raw sugar or dress it up with maple sugar crystals.

TIP Warming the milk makes these cakes creamier.

PER SERVING› Energy 69 cal, **Fat** 3 g, **Sodium** 116 mg, **Carbs** 8 g, **Fiber** 0 g, **Protein** 3 g, **Water** 63%

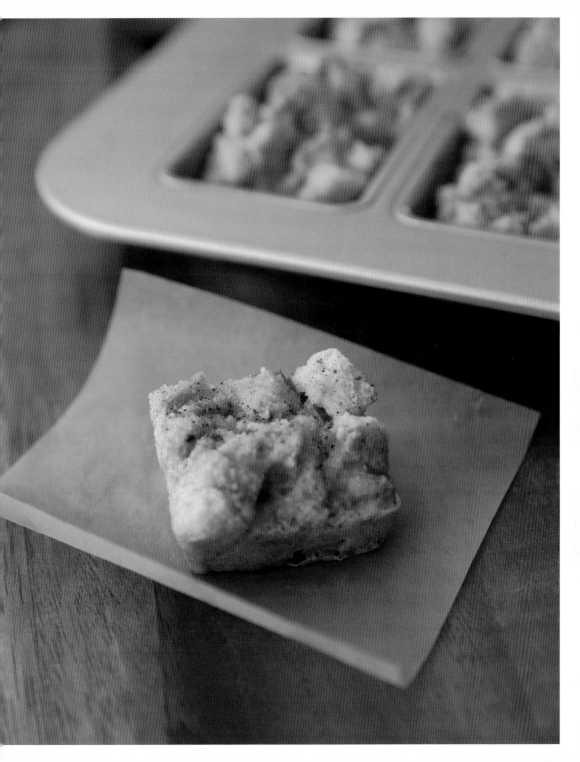

CHOCOLATE CAKES

4 eggs + 1 egg yolk

¾ cup almond milk, heated

2 tablespoons melted butter
or coconut oil

1 tablespoon brown sugar

2 tablespoons unsweetened
cocoa powder

1 teaspoon vanilla extract

½ teaspoon ground cinnamon

4 cups cubed gluten-free bread,
tightly packed (~half a loaf)

½ cup semisweet
chocolate chips, melted

Heat oven to 350 degrees. Lightly coat a muffin tin or an 8" square baking pan with nonstick cooking spray.

Place the eggs and egg yolk in a small food processor and pulse a few times.

Warm the almond milk in the microwave on high for 1 minute. Add the milk, melted butter, brown sugar, cocoa, vanilla, and cinnamon into the food processor and pulse until fully incorporated.

Add bread cubes and let soak for a few minutes. For a smooth batter, pulse the cake batter once more to break down the bread cubes. Fold in the chocolate chips.

Pour the batter into the pan. If using a muffin tin, fill each form ¾ full.

Bake in a muffin tin for 12–15 minutes, baking pan for 30 minutes, or until a toothpick inserted into the center comes out clean.

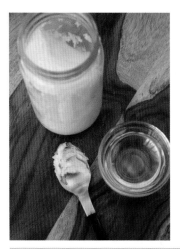

VIRGIN COCONUT OIL is a sweet vegetable fat with a light vanilla flavor. While higher in saturated fat, it's unrefined and generally thought to be easier to digest and less harmful than other saturated fats. Use coconut oil as a substitute for butter.

PER SERVING› Energy 107 cal, **Fat** 6 g, **Sodium** 108 mg, **Carbs** 12 g, **Fiber** 1 g, **Protein** 3 g, **Water** 30%

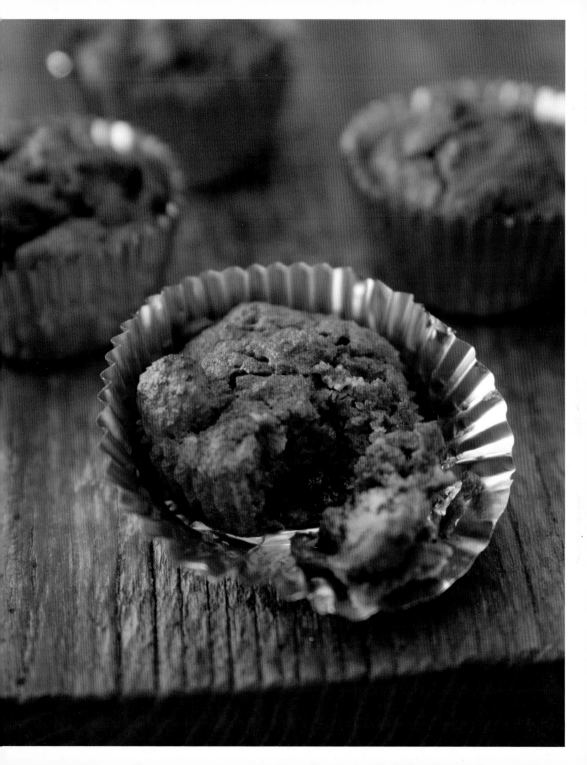

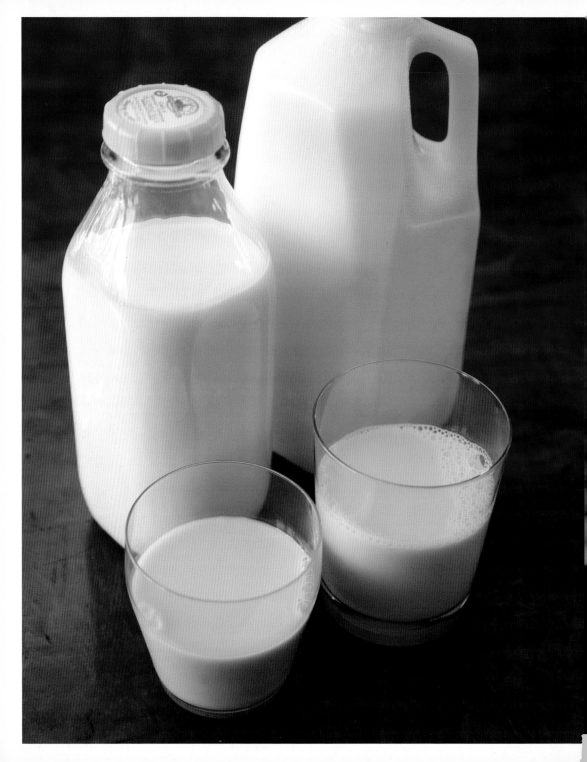

MILK: USE WHAT YOU'VE GOT

We have specified a particular milk variety in most of our recipes, but you can use whatever you tolerate best or have on hand. Try out different milks to find the flavor you prefer.

Soy milk has a nutty flavor and a somewhat gritty texture. Higher in protein and carbs, it packs in the calories. Rice milk offers a mild flavor with plenty of carbs, and no protein. Almond milk has a bit more fragrance and a rich, nutty flavor lower in carbs and protein. Similar from a nutritional standpoint, coconut milk (not to be confused with canned coconut milk) is thick and smooth with mildly sweet flavor and a bit more fat. Dairy milk has a mild, cheesy flavor and a robust nutritional profile.

INGREDIENT› ½ CUP	ENERGY (CAL)	FAT (G)	SODIUM (MG)	CARB (G)	FIBER (G)	PROTEIN (G)	WATER (%)
Dairy, 1%	51	1	54	6	–	4	90
Dairy, 2%	61	3	50	6	–	4	89
Dairy, skim/nonfat	43	–	64	6	–	4	91
Dairy, whole	73	4	49	6	–	4	89
Almond, unsweetened	20	2	90	1	–	1	92
Coconut, unsweetened	25	3	8	1	–	1	92
Soy, unsweetened	52	1	40	8	–	4	92
Rice, unsweetened	35	1	62	6	–	–	92

TIP LOW-FAT DAIRY MILK will be thinner than other varieties, so you might need to adjust the recipe slightly to get the right consistency.

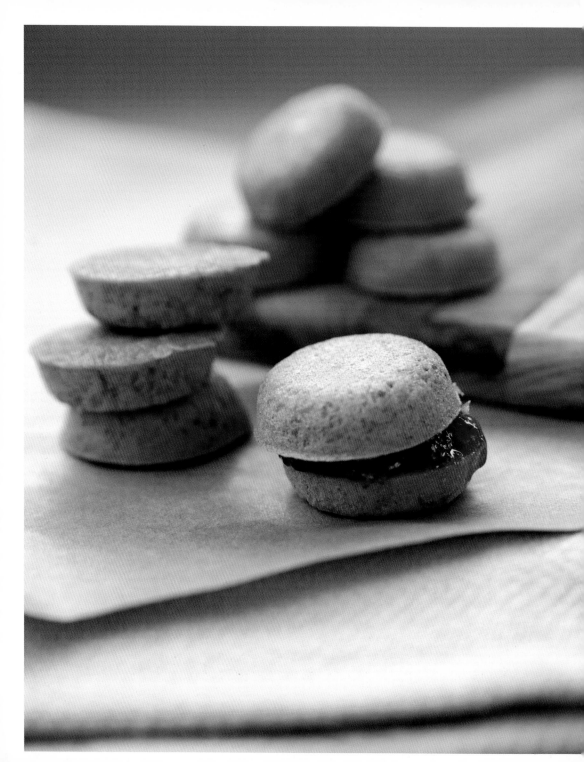

SERVINGS> 12
TIME> 5 minutes prep,
40 minutes in oven

SPICED PUMPKIN CAKES

5 eggs + 1 egg yolk

½ cup cooked pumpkin
(canned or prepared at home)

¼ cup soy milk

2 tablespoons melted butter
or coconut oil

1 teaspoon vanilla extract

1 tablespoon brown sugar

1 teaspoon ground cinnamon

½ teaspoon ground nutmeg

½ teaspoon salt

4 cups cubed gluten-free bread,
tightly packed (~half a loaf)

Heat oven to 350 degrees. Lightly coat a muffin tin or 8" square baking pan with nonstick cooking spray.

In a blender or small food processor, mix together eggs, egg yolk, pumpkin, milk, and melted butter and process for a minute or two until the eggs lighten.

Add vanilla, brown sugar, cinnamon, nutmeg, and salt and pulse to incorporate.

Fold in bread cubes and let soak for 5 minutes. Pulse the mixture until it becomes a smooth batter. The batter will be thin. Spoon mixture into a muffin tin.

Bake for 15–20 minutes or until a toothpick inserted into the center comes out clean. (If using mini muffin tins, bake 8–10 minutes.)

Makes 24 mini muffins (2 per serving) or 12 standard muffins.

TIP We made these pumpkin cakes in a **MINI MUFFIN TIN**, so we pureed the batter to make a smooth cake. Use whatever baking pan you have on hand, and whether chunky or smooth, you will find these pumpkin bites irresistible.

PER SERVING> Energy 108 cal, **Fat** 6 g, **Sodium** 230 mg, **Carbs** 10 g, **Fiber** 1 g, **Protein** 4 g, **Water** 45%

SWEET CREAM GRITS

4 cups water

2 cups uncooked grits

3 egg yolks, lightly beaten

2 tablespoons raw sugar

1 teaspoon vanilla extract

Cream of Wheat is a great alternative to grits, but it does contain gluten.

Lightly coat a muffin tin or ramekins with nonstick cooking spray.

Bring water with a dash of salt to a boil in a saucepan over high heat. Add grits, stirring frequently for 3–4 minutes. Remove from heat to add egg yolks. Return to heat and simmer on low until mixture thickens, then stir in raw sugar and vanilla.

Pour cooked grits into muffin cups or ramekins and let set for 10–15 minutes to firm up.

TIP › Serve up your grits like CRÈME BRÛLÉE: Top with additional raw sugar and place under the broiler until the sugar turns brown. Let cool before handling.

PER SERVING› Energy 113 cal, **Fat** 1 g, **Sodium** 14 mg, **Carbs** 22 g, **Fiber** 0 g, **Protein** 3 g, **Water** 61%

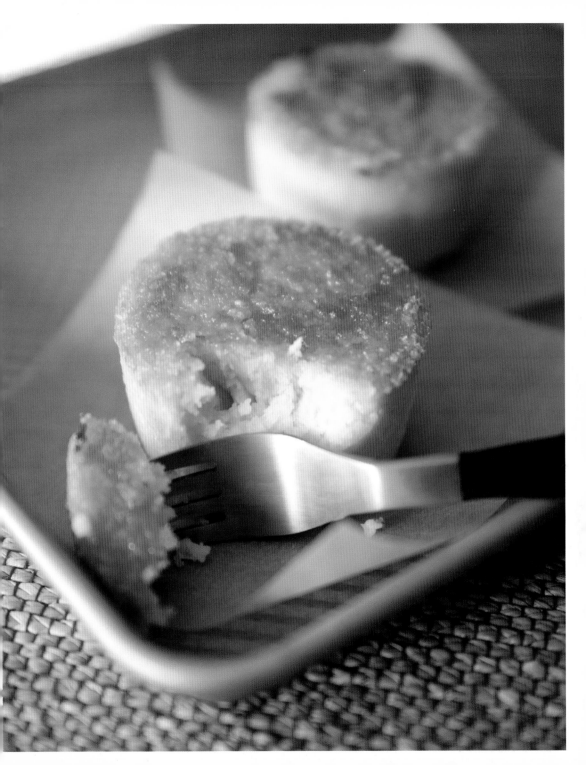

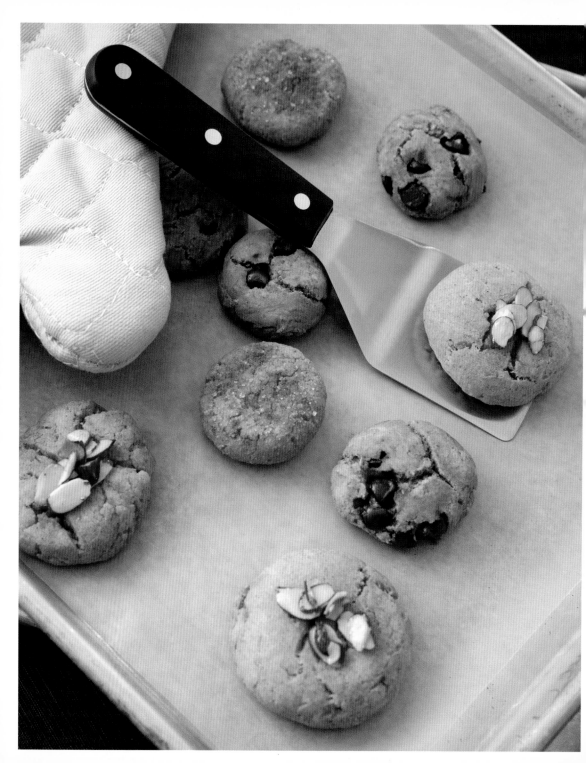

SERVINGS› 12
TIME› 5 minutes prep,
15 minutes in oven

COOKIES

These dense, slightly chewy cookies have become a training camp favorite. You can find any number of delicious gluten-free cookie recipes, but they are complicated with lots of expensive ingredients. We've simplified these to include ingredients that you will be able to use with other recipes in this book.

SNICKERDOODLE COOKIES

1 cup brown rice flour

2 tablespoons potato flour

2 tablespoons brown sugar

¼ teaspoon baking powder

¼ teaspoon coarse salt

¼ teaspoon cream of tartar

½ cup soy or almond milk, heated

1 tablespoon coconut oil or butter

1 egg

½ teaspoon vanilla extract

TOP IT OFF

2 tablespoons raw sugar + 1 teaspoon ground cinnamon

NUT BUTTER COOKIES

1 cup brown rice flour

¼ cup potato flour

2 teaspoons brown sugar

¼ teaspoon baking powder

¼ teaspoon coarse salt

¾ cup almond milk, heated

¼ cup almond butter ← *Use whatever nuts and nut butter you have on hand.*

½ teaspoon vanilla extract

TOP IT OFF

2 tablespoons sliced almonds

TIP Add up to 2 tablespoons of apple sauce or plain yogurt if you like your cookies **EXTRA MOIST**. The finish will vary a bit depending on your oven and the humidity and elevation where you live.

PER SERVING

Snickerdoodle› **Energy** 84 cal, **Fat** 2 g, **Sodium** 64 mg, **Carbs** 15 g, **Fiber** 1 g, **Protein** 2 g, **Water** 33%
Nut Butter› **Energy** 93 cal, **Fat** 4 g, **Sodium** 84 mg, **Carbs** 15 g, **Fiber** 1 g, **Protein** 2 g, **Water** 31%

CHOCOLATE CHIP COOKIES

1 cup brown rice flour

2 tablespoons potato flour

1 tablespoon brown sugar

1 teaspoon unsweetened cocoa powder

¼ teaspoon baking powder

¼ teaspoon coarse salt

½ cup almond milk, heated

1 tablespoon coconut oil

1 egg

½ teaspoon vanilla extract

¼ cup semisweet chocolate chips

TOP IT OFF

2 tablespoons raw sugar + 1 tablespoon coarse salt

TO MAKE COOKIES

Heat oven to 350 degrees. Lightly coat a baking sheet with nonstick cooking spray or line with parchment paper.

In a large bowl, combine the dry ingredients.

Heat the milk for 90 seconds in the microwave, or until very hot. Add the coconut oil or butter to the hot milk to melt it (nut butter cookies don't require oil). Quickly whisk in the egg or almond butter and any other wet ingredients.

Pour the hot mixture into the bowl of dry ingredients. Stir until thoroughly combined. ⟵

If applicable, fold in the chocolate chips.

Set the dough aside to cool for a moment as you prepare the topping. Shape cookies into 12 golf-ball size balls, lightly flatten, and top with a generous pinch of sugar-cinnamon, nuts, or sugar-salt. You will have topping left over.

Bake for 15 minutes.

Let cool and store cookies in the fridge in an airtight container for up to 3 days. Keep the cookies separated or they might stick together.

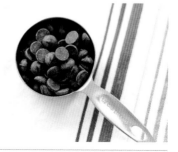

PER SERVING

Chocolate Chip› Energy 91 cal, **Fat** 3 g, **Sodium** 116 mg, **Carbs** 15 g, **Fiber** 1 g, **Protein** 2 g, **Water** 43%

Cooking real food doesn't have to be an all-out chore. ★ Like most things worth doing *it just needs to be practiced and planned for*.

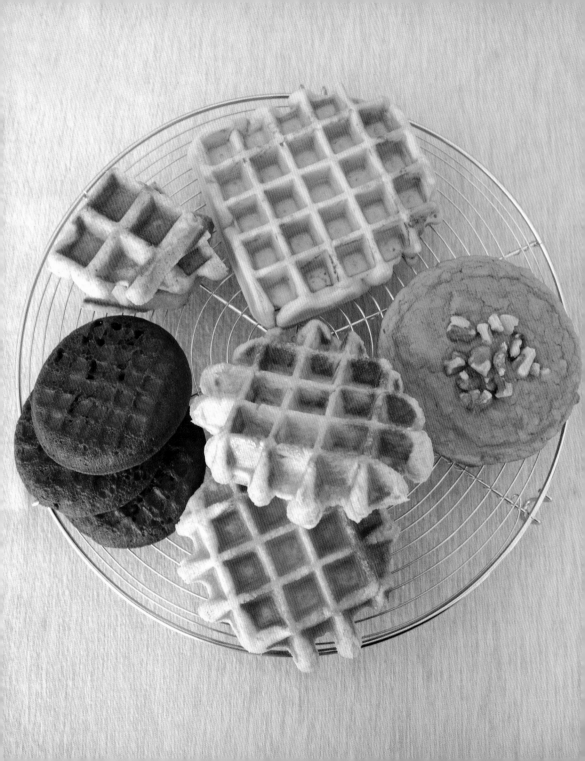

GRIDDLE CAKES, PANCAKES & WAFFLES

These are some of the most portable foods around. Wrap up a small stack or make up sandwiches with a combination of meat, cheese, nut butter, and spreads. Waffles are especially great at tucking away more flavor without a mess.

Don't have a waffle iron? Don't let that stop you. Pour the batter right into a sauté pan or griddle, or experiment with different types of baking pans.

We've kept the batches small in case you're cooking for one or two, but you can double any of these recipes to stock the freezer with your favorite variety.

V VEGETARIAN   G GLUTEN-FREE

WAFFLE AND PANCAKE BATTERS can be prepared a number of different ways. For a more hands-free option, we baked up some of these pancake recipes in the oven using whoopie pie and tart pans. Be creative to find the option that works best for you. Simply refer to the cooking grid below for approximate cooking/baking times.

METHOD	TIME	NOTES
Pancakes (griddle/stovetop)	10–15 minutes	Makes 10–12 pancakes or 6 servings.
Tarts (baking sheet)	15–20 minutes	Heat oven to 400 degrees. Makes 4 large tarts.
Waffle iron	8–10 minutes*	Makes 4 large waffles. Cut into 8 sandwiches.
Whoopie pie (baking sheet)	10–12 minutes	Makes 12 thin "pies." Makes 6 sandwiches.

*Cooking time will vary depending on the size of your waffle iron. A full size waffle iron cooks up 4 waffles at a time, which is a full batch for most of the recipes. Review the instructions that accompanied the waffle iron for additional cooking tips.

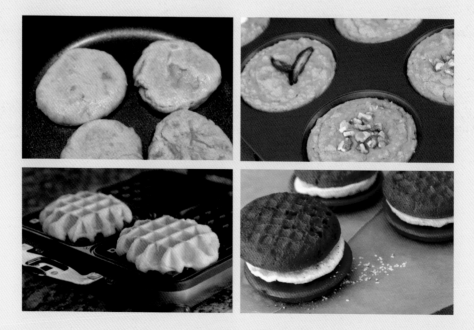

★ ★ ★

"Pancakes are my personal favorite. My diet doesn't have to be boring or austere to go fast. In fact, I go way faster when I'm happy, and good food makes me happy."

LEA DAVISON
OLYMPIAN, CROSS-COUNTRY
3RD, NATIONAL CHAMPIONSHIPS,
SHORT TRACK

GRIDDLE CAKES

1½ cups all-purpose flour

½ teaspoon sugar

1 cup almond milk, heated

¼ teaspoon cinnamon (optional)

You can substitute gluten-free baking mix or masa harina for all-purpose flour.

Heat oven to 350 degrees. Brush a sauté pan or griddle lightly with vegetable or canola oil and bring to medium-high heat.

Combine the flour and sugar in a medium bowl and stir together.

Add cinnamon here if using.

Heat the almond milk in the microwave for 90 seconds and pour it into the dry mixture. Quickly stir it in with a wooden spoon. Once the dough begins to hold together, work it with your hands until all of the flour is incorporated. Divide the dough into 6 portions, each rolled a little larger than a golf ball.

Using the palm of your hand, flatten each ball of dough to be about ¼-inch thick. Fry on the griddle until golden brown on both sides, approximately 3 minutes per side.

Finish in the oven for 5 minutes to cook the centers.

Let cakes cool before wrapping.

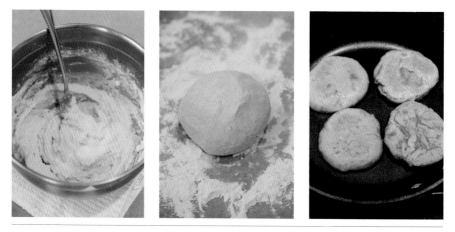

PER SERVING› Energy 128 cal, **Fat** 1 g, **Sodium** 26 mg, **Carbs** 26 g, **Fiber** 1 g, **Protein** 3 g, **Water** 27%

The **WARM DOUGH** we use to make our stuffed two-bite pies is equally great on the griddle. This is a very basic recipe that can be expanded in countless ways, but we love the simplicity of these cakes—eat them piping hot with jam or honey.

SCALLION PANCAKES

1 cup flour

½ teaspoon salt

4 chopped scallions or green onions (green parts only)

½ cup boiling water

1 tablespoon sesame oil

You can substitute vegetable or canola oil for sesame oil.

Combine the flour, salt, and scallions in a medium bowl and stir together.

Pour the boiling water over the dry mixture. Quickly stir it with a wooden spoon. Once the dough begins to hold together, work it with your hands until all of the flour is incorporated. Shape the dough into a large ball.

On a lightly floured surface, roll the dough into a circle about ⅛-inch thick, similar to a tortilla.

Brush a sauté pan with sesame oil and bring to medium-high heat. Fry the pancake on the griddle until golden brown on both sides, about 3 minutes per side.

Cut into 8 wedges (2 per serving). Let cool before wrapping.

TIP If you use sesame oil, bring the pan to heat slowly so the oil doesn't smoke you out of the kitchen.

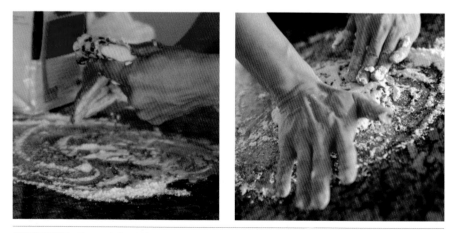

PER SERVING› Energy 145 cal, **Fat** 4 g, **Sodium** 293 mg, **Carbs** 24 g, **Fiber** 1 g, **Protein** 3 g, **Water** 43%

This is a **CHINESE-STYLE PANCAKE**, savory in flavor, and crispier and thinner than the Western variety.

POTATO FLAKES are a portables staple and the fastest way to pack in some carbs at home or on the road. Check the ingredients— a quality brand will simply list dehydrated potatoes.

MASHED POTATO CAKES

1 cup instant potato flakes

2 tablespoons grated parmesan

COOKED 2 tablespoons chopped cooked bacon

1 tablespoon minced fresh tarragon

1 vegetable bouillon cube

1½ cups hot water

2 eggs, lightly beaten

Brush a griddle lightly with vegetable or canola oil and bring to medium-high heat.

Combine potato flakes, parmesan, bacon, and tarragon in a medium bowl.

Dissolve bouillon in hot water before adding to the potato flake mixture. Add eggs and quickly stir until the potato flakes are incorporated. Batter will be thick and somewhat lumpy.

Spoon batter onto the griddle, forming small cakes. Cook until golden brown, about 5–6 minutes per side.

Makes 10–12 small cakes (2–3 per serving). Let cakes cool before wrapping.

TIP If you have an electric griddle or hot plate, these cakes will travel. Simply combine the dry ingredients in a ziplock bag (omit the bacon and substitute ¼ teaspoon of your favorite dried herb for the fresh tarragon).

PER SERVING› Energy 125 cal, **Fat** 5 g, **Sodium** 349mg, **Carbs** 13 g, **Fiber** 1 g, **Protein** 6 g, **Water** 70%

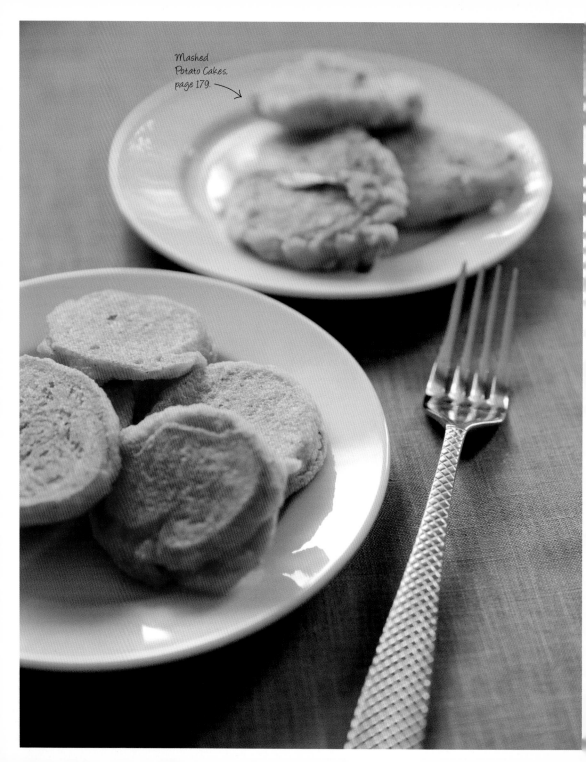

Mashed
Potato Cakes,
page 179.

SWEET CORN CAKES

1 cup masa harina

¼ cup raw sugar

2 tablespoons brown rice flour

¼ teaspoon baking powder

½ teaspoon ground cinnamon

dash of coarse salt

1 egg, lightly beaten

2 tablespoons melted butter or softened coconut oil

1 cup soy milk, heated

Brush a griddle lightly with vegetable or canola oil and bring to medium-high heat.

Combine dry ingredients in a large bowl. Add egg and butter or coconut oil and mix well.

Heat the soy milk for 90 seconds in the microwave. Quickly stir it into the mixture to fully melt the coconut oil. Let the batter rest for a few minutes to thicken before cooking.

Spoon the batter onto the griddle, forming small cakes. Cook until golden brown, about 3 minutes per side.

Makes 10–12 small cakes (2–3 per serving). Let cakes cool before wrapping.

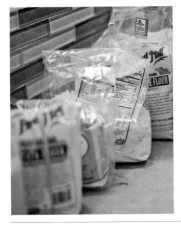

MASA HARINA is a flour used to make corn tortillas and is available in the Mexican food aisle at most grocers.

PER SERVING› Energy 276 cal, **Fat** 10 g, **Sodium** 95 mg, **Carbs** 42 g, **Fiber** 3 g, **Protein** 6 g, **Water** 47%

The **MILD FLAVOR** of these waffles goes well with savory or sweet spreads.

CARROT WAFFLES

1 cup flour

1 tablespoon raw sugar

¼ teaspoon baking powder

pinch of salt

½ cup fresh carrot juice

2 eggs, lightly beaten

2 tablespoons melted butter

½ cup carrot pulp (optional)

Heat the waffle iron.

Mix dry ingredients together in a medium bowl. In a separate bowl or measuring cup, combine carrot juice, eggs, and melted butter.

Add wet ingredients to the dry mixture and whisk together until flour is thoroughly incorporated. ← *Add carrot pulp here if using.* The batter will be a bit lumpy.

Pour enough batter into each waffle form to nearly fill all the squares (the batter will expand when pressed). Cook until the outside of the waffle feels crisp to the touch. Repeat if necessary, using remaining batter.

Makes 4 large waffles. Let cool, then cut in half and stack for easy wrapping.

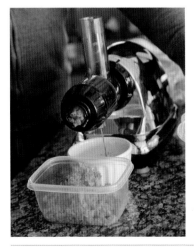

For great texture and a boost in fiber, try adding **PULP** to the waffle batter.

PER SERVING› Energy 223 cal, **Fat** 9 g, **Sodium** 75 mg, **Carbs** 30 g, **Fiber** 1 g, **Protein** 7 g, **Water** 41%

BEET JUICE WAFFLE SANDWICHES

1 cup flour

1 tablespoon raw sugar

¼ teaspoon baking powder

pinch of salt

½ cup fresh beet juice

2 eggs, lightly beaten

1 tablespoon molasses

2 tablespoons melted butter

½ cup beet pulp (optional)

*You can substitute pomegranate juice
for beet juice if you don't have a juicer.*

Heat oven to 350 degrees. Lightly coat a whoopie
pie baking pan with nonstick cooking spray.

Mix dry ingredients together in a medium bowl.
In a bowl or measuring cup, blend together beet
juice, eggs, molasses, and melted butter.

Add wet ingredients to the dry mixture and whisk ← *Add beet pulp here if using.*
together until flour is thoroughly incorporated.
The batter will be a bit lumpy.

Use a small measuring cup to fill each whoopie pie
form. Bake for 10–12 minutes, or until the centers
are set.

*Makes 12 whoopie pies, which can be stacked into
6 sandwiches.*

PER SERVING › Energy 160 cal, **Fat** 6 g, **Sodium** 84 mg, **Carbs** 23 g, **Fiber** 1 g, **Protein** 4 g, **Water** 50%

With **BEET JUICE AND MOLASSES,** these waffles have an Old World flavor that goes great with poached eggs or as an accompaniment to a hearty roasted dinner.

Choose products and recipes with a *minimal number of ingredients*, preferably real food, that you can recognize and that don't challenge your intelligence even if they challenge your desire for convenience and insult a massive industry selling us quantity over quality.

★ ★ ★

"Allen and Biju introduced me to the concept of eating real food in triathlon training and racing and it has made all of the difference. Using portables on the bike, I can head out onto the run feeling fueled and ready to race hard to the finish."

KRISTEN PETERSON
RÊVE TOUR, TOUR DE FRANCE
AQUATHLON NATIONAL CHAMPION

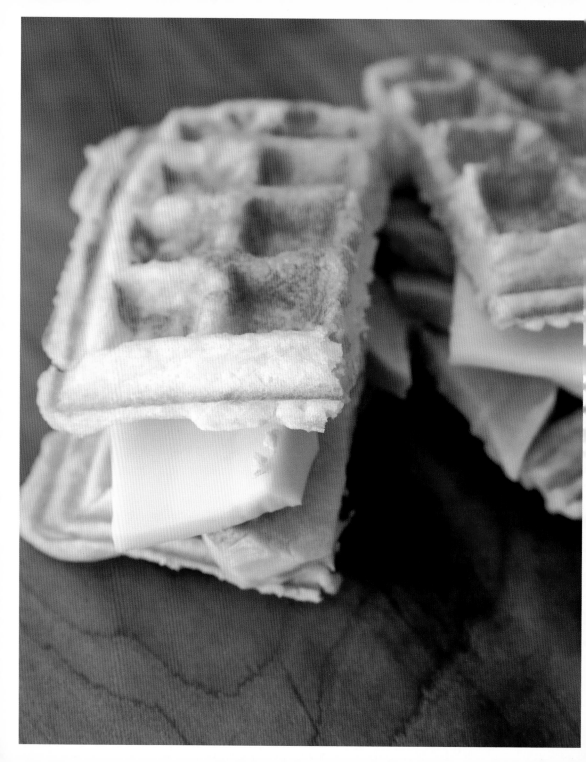

CHEESY POTATO WAFFLES

¾ cup potato flakes

¼ cup potato flour

¼ cup brown rice flour

2 tablespoons grated parmesan

½ teaspoon salt

½ teaspoon baking powder

1 cup almond milk, heated

4 eggs, lightly beaten

Heat the waffle iron.

Combine the potato flakes with the flours, cheese, salt, and baking powder in a large bowl.

Heat the almond milk in the microwave on high for 90 seconds. Add the milk and the eggs to the dry mixture and stir until the potato flakes and flours are fully incorporated. Batter will be dense and somewhat lumpy.

Pour enough batter into each waffle form to nearly fill all the squares (the batter will expand when pressed). Cook until the outside of the waffle feels crisp to the touch. Repeat, using remaining batter.

Makes 4 large waffles. Let cool, then cut in half and stack for easy wrapping.

PER SERVING> Energy 230 cal, **Fat** 8 g, **Sodium** 567 mg, **Carbs** 31 g, **Fiber** 2 g, **Protein** 10 g, **Water** 35%

BANANA WAFFLES

1 cup cubed gluten-free bread, tightly packed

½ cup white rice flour

¼ cup ground almonds

pinch of ground nutmeg

1 tablespoon brown sugar

2 eggs, lightly beaten

¼ cup almond milk

1 large ripe banana

Heat the waffle iron.

Place the dry ingredients in a food processor and pulse quickly to combine.

In a small bowl or measuring cup, combine the eggs and almond milk and stir briskly. Pour this into the food processor, add the banana, and pulse. Batter should be smooth and somewhat dense.

Pour enough batter into each waffle form to nearly fill all the squares (the batter will expand when pressed). Cook until the outside of the waffle feels crisp. Repeat, using the remaining batter.

Makes 4 large waffles. Cut each waffle into quarters and top with your favorite spread(s) to make 8 mini waffle sandwiches. Let cool before wrapping.

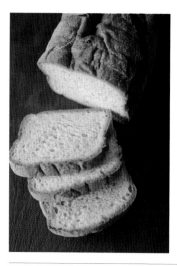

In a recipe like this one, **GLUTEN-FREE BREAD** shortcuts some of the extra flours and makes for a unique texture. The water content of bread is somewhat lower than other carbs, though 43 percent is still well above pre-packaged foods.

PER SERVING › Energy 112 cal, Fat 3 g, Sodium 60 mg, Carbs 17 g, Fiber 1 g, Protein 4 g, Water 43%

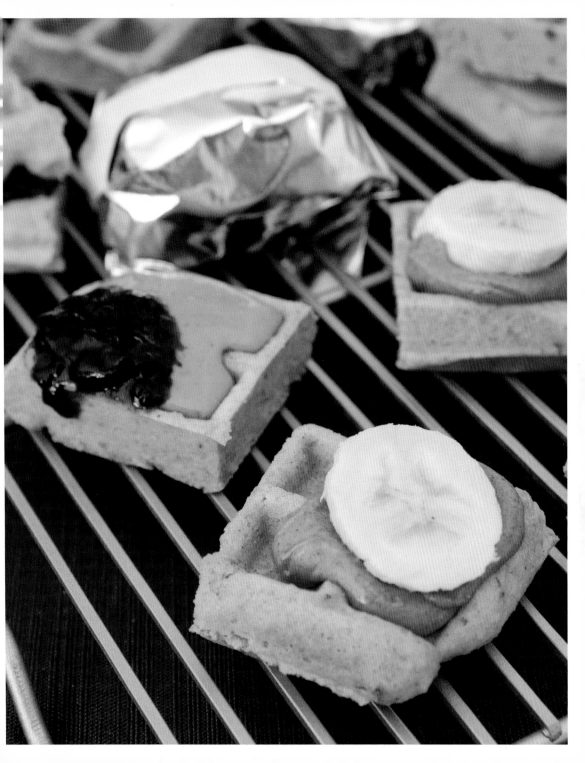

As a general rule of thumb, when you're in a period when you're not training or are training very little, it's okay to be hungry. ★ When you are training, be a little hungry. ★ And when you're getting close to a major competition or even when you are competing, make sure that you aren't hungry.

SPREADS like classic nut butters, cream cheese, and preserves turn your waffles into fun and easy portables for those long rides.

SWEET POTATO CAKES

2 medium sweet potatoes,
peeled and cubed

2 eggs

2 tablespoons melted butter

2 tablespoons maple syrup

¼ cup brown rice flour

½ teaspoon ground cinnamon

dash of salt

COOKED 1 cup cooked rice

Heat the oven to 400 degrees. Lightly coat a tart baking sheet with nonstick cooking spray.

Cook the cubed sweet potatoes in the microwave until fork-tender, about 3 to 5 minutes.

Place the sweet potatoes, eggs, butter, and maple syrup in a food processor and pulse until mixture is smooth.

Add the flour, cinnamon, and salt to the mixture and pulse until fully incorporated.

Finally, add the rice, taking care not to overprocess— simply pulse to work the rice into the batter or stir it in by hand. Batter will be thick.

Use a small measuring cup to fill each tart form. Bake for 15–20 minutes, or until the centers are set.

The cooked rice gives these cakes a rich, custard-like texture. Top with your favorite chopped nuts and let them set up for at least 10–15 minutes or in the refrigerator overnight.

TIP This recipe can also make 6 delicious waffles. Allow some extra time for the thick batter to cook fully.

PER SERVING› Energy 259 cal, **Fat** 9 g, **Sodium** 98 mg, **Carbs** 39 g, **Fiber** 3 g, **Protein** 6 g, **Water** 56%

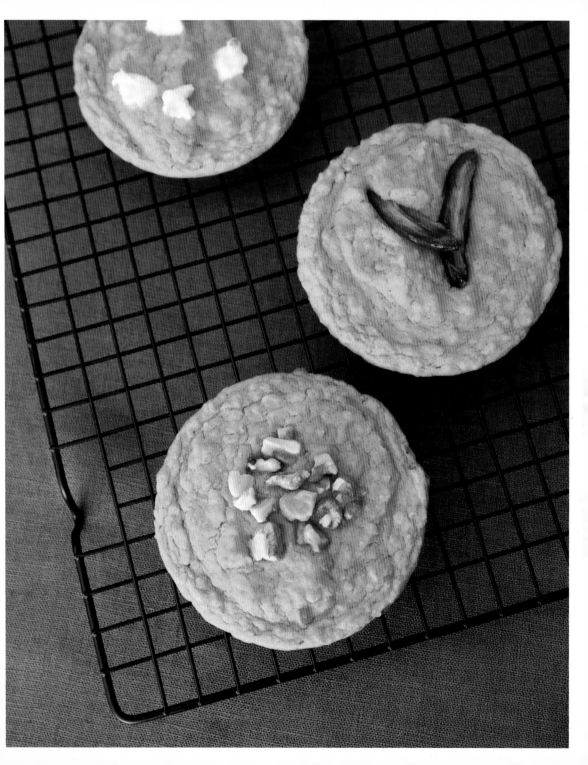

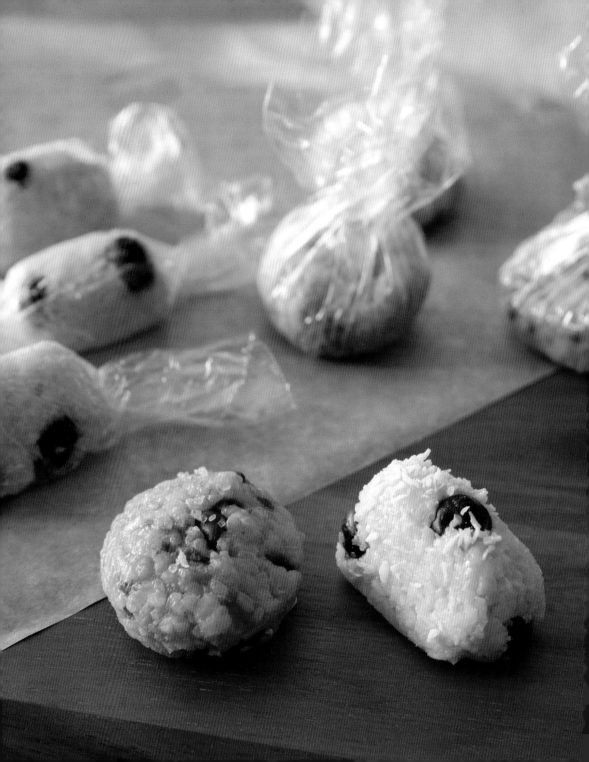

AHA! PORTABLES

"Aha!" portables begin with common, everyday foods that you most likely have on hand. With a little ingenuity, these foods can be reinvented to be easy and convenient to take along on a long training ride.

Be creative as you make your own rice balls, rolled breads, baked pastas, and sticky bites. Use whatever shapes you can find to create a small, packed portable. As you will see, we've used everything from espresso cups to ice cube trays.

We hope that by showing you some variations on the same theme, we can inspire you to come up with a few aha! portables of your own.

★★★

"I've eaten all sorts of things on the bike—boiled potatoes rolled in salt and parmesan, slices of pizza, cookies, muffins, banana breads. I once got on a black licorice kick. I love experimenting with new foods and flavors on the bike."

LUCAS EUSER
UNITED HEALTHCARE PRO CYCLING TEAM
1ST, UCI 2.1 UNIVEST GRAND PRIX

V VEGETARIAN   **G** GLUTEN-FREE

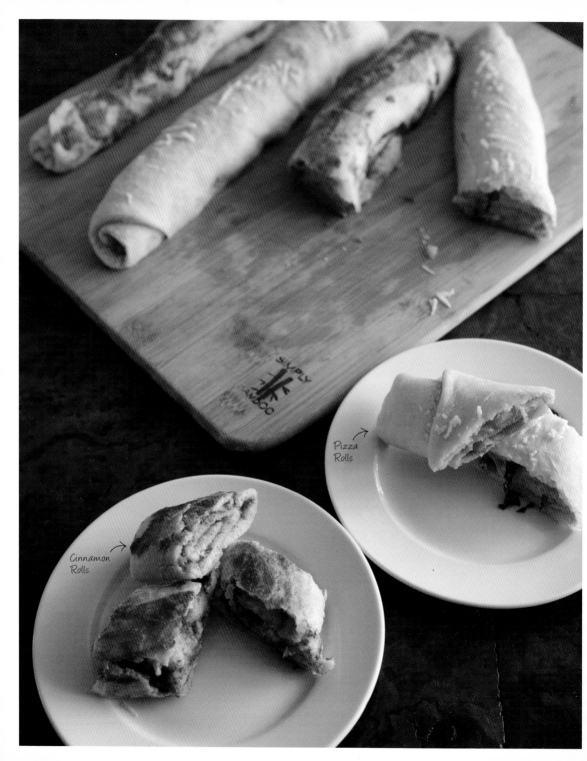

Pizza
Rolls

Cinnamon
Rolls

SAVORY & SWEET ROLLS

Here are portable takes on two popular favorites—pizza and cinnamon rolls. There's no shortage of pizzerias and bakeries in Europe, so it's only natural that cyclists would find reason to stop for a sweet bread treat or rolled up slice of margherita pizza in the middle of a long training ride. Simply go easy on the fillings and you can enjoy the flavors you love without a mess (or indigestion).

PIZZA ROLLS

½ batch Basic Dough
(recipe on page 203)

2 tablespoons pizza sauce

1 tablespoon shredded mozzarella

1 tablespoon chopped fresh basil

1 tablespoon chopped prosciutto

TOP WITH
olive oil + sprinkle of coarse salt

CINNAMON ROLLS

½ batch Basic Dough
(recipe on page 203)

4 tablespoons butter, melted

2 tablespoons brown sugar + 1 teaspoon ground cinnamon

1 tablespoon dried currants

TOP WITH
remaining butter + sprinkle of raw sugar

TIP Once baked, these rolls can be cut into bite-size portions, individually wrapped, and kept in the FREEZER.

TO MAKE SAVORY & SWEET ROLLS

Heat oven to 375 degrees. Lightly coat a baking pan with nonstick cooking spray or line with parchment paper.

Using a rolling pin or wine bottle, roll out half of the dough into an oblong shape, approximately 8" × 12", just under ¼" thick. Flip it once or twice, stretching the dough from the center outward.

Spread just enough melted butter or pizza sauce to lightly cover the dough. Too much gets messy. Top evenly with remaining ingredients.

Roll up the dough lengthwise and gently pinch the edge to seal. Transfer bread roll to the baking sheet. Repeat with the rest of the dough to make the second bread roll.

Lightly brush the top of the roll with melted butter or olive oil. Sprinkle with sugar or salt. Bake for 15 minutes or until the bread is golden.

Cut each roll into 12 small portions.

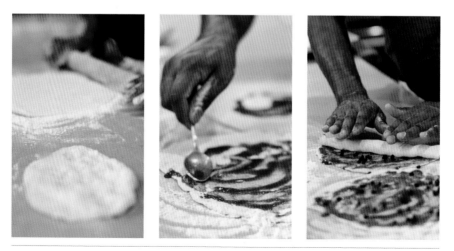

PER SERVING
Pizza Rolls› Energy 72 cal, **Fat** 1 g, **Sodium** 198 mg, **Carbs** 13 g, **Fiber** 1 g, **Protein** 2 g, **Water** 35%
Cinnamon Rolls› Energy 114 cal, **Fat** 5 g, **Sodium** 84 mg, **Carbs** 16 g, **Fiber** 1 g, **Protein** 2 g, **Water** 25%

BASIC DOUGH

This recipe makes enough dough for two bread rolls, so you can have it all—savory and sweet.

1 cup warm tap water

1 tablespoon active dry yeast

½ teaspoon sugar

3 cups all-purpose flour,
plus more for rolling dough

2 tablespoons olive oil or butter

1 teaspoon coarse salt

In a large bowl combine water, yeast, and sugar, and gently mix. Set aside for about 5 minutes or until the mixture is foamy.

Stir in 2½ cups flour, 1 tablespoon of the olive oil or butter, and the salt. Dough will be sticky.

Transfer dough to a floured surface and knead while adding remaining ½ cup flour in small amounts until you get a consistent, nonsticky, elastic dough.

Coat another large bowl with the remaining olive oil. Place dough in bowl, turning to coat evenly with oil. Cover with a damp cloth and let rise in a warm place until dough has doubled in size, about 1 hour. If you are not prepping the dough right away, cover it with plastic wrap and store in the refrigerator.

Makes 2 batches of rolls (24 servings).

TIP Most natural grocery stores sell **FRESH OR FROZEN DOUGH** with minimal ingredients. Check your local store to cut your bread roll prep in half.

PER SERVING› Energy 68 cal, **Fat** 1 g, **Sodium** 83 mg, **Carbs** 13 g, **Fiber** 1 g, **Protein** 2 g, **Water** 32%

BAKED PASTA

1 pound uncooked
thin spaghetti

1 cup chopped pancetta
or bacon

8 eggs

¼ cup chopped fresh basil

2 tablespoons grated parmesan

Small pasta like elbow macaroni or penne will work in this dish too.

Heat oven to 350 degrees. Lightly coat a muffin tin with nonstick cooking spray.

Bring a large pot of water to a boil. Add the pasta and cook for 6–8 minutes, or until al dente, drain and set aside.

While the pasta is boiling, cook the pancetta in a sauté pan over medium-high heat until crisp. Drain fat and set aside.

In a large bowl, lightly beat the eggs. Mix in the pancetta and basil, and then fold in the pasta.

Use tongs to keep turning the pasta so the egg and meat are evenly distributed as you generously fill the muffin tins (the pasta will not expand when it bakes). Sprinkle with cheese and bake for 12–15 minutes, or until the egg has fully set. (Be careful not to overbake—the noodles will become crunchy and difficult to chew.)

While the pan is still warm, use a disposable knife to loosen the pasta from the muffin forms. Let cool before wrapping. Store baked pasta in the fridge for up to 3 days.

PER SERVING› Energy 135 cal, **Fat** 5 g, **Sodium** 122 mg, **Carbs** 14 g, **Fiber** 1 g, **Protein** 8 g, **Water** 39%

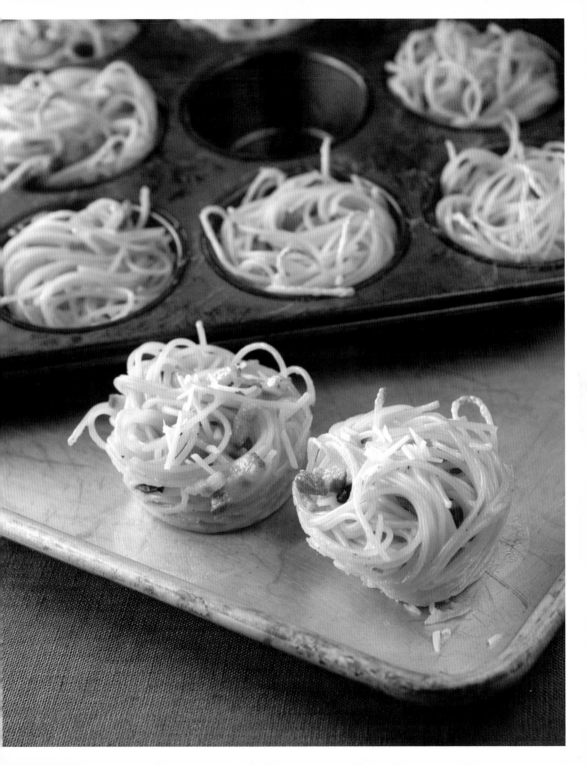

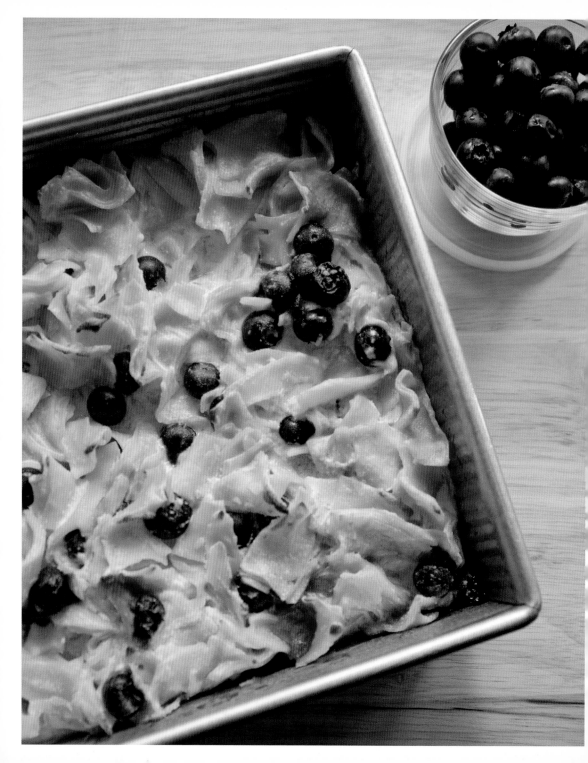

BLUEBERRY KUGEL

This Jewish holiday treat happens to be a mix of all our favorite ingredients. I adapted the traditional recipe by substituting yogurt for sour cream, decreasing the number of eggs, and keeping the flavors very mild.

8 ounces wide egg noodles

½ cup ricotta cheese

½ cup plain Greek yogurt

2 eggs, lightly beaten

¼ cup milk

2 tablespoons brown sugar

½ teaspoon vanilla extract

1 cup fresh blueberries

You can substitute palm or coconut sugar for brown sugar.

Heat oven to 375 degrees. Lightly coat an 8" or 9" square baking pan with nonstick cooking spray.

In a large saucepan bring water with a dash of salt to a boil and cook the egg noodles until al dente. Strain and set aside.

Combine the cheese, yogurt, eggs, milk, sugar, and vanilla in a large bowl, mixing until all ingredients are incorporated.

Gently fold in the blueberries and cooked egg noodles.

Transfer the mixture to the baking pan. Loosely cover with foil and bake for 30 minutes, then remove cover and continue to bake for another 10 minutes or until the kugel is firm and the top is beginning to brown. (Be careful not to overbake—the noodles will become crunchy and difficult to chew.)

Let cool before cutting. The flavor is best when you let the kugel set in the fridge for a few hours or overnight.

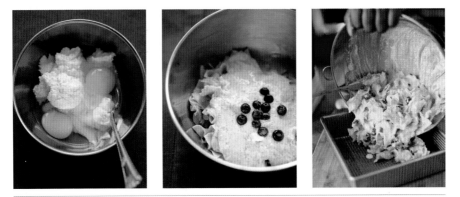

PER SERVING› Energy 129 cal, **Fat** 0 g, **Sodium** 31 mg, **Carbs** 18 g, **Fiber** 1 g, **Protein** 6 g, **Water** 35%

"Having personally handed out hundreds of *Feed Zone* rice cakes to some of the best athletes on the planet, I can attest that there is a direct correlation between these portables and improved performance and recovery. Simply put, this is very healthy, creative food developed by smart people who care . . . and the taste is sublime!"

DAVIS PHINNEY
OLYMPIC BRONZE MEDALIST, TEAM TIME TRIAL
USPRO NATIONAL CHAMPION
2-TIME TOUR DE FRANCE STAGE WINNER

Managing the intake of food and drink using recipes, real foods, and products that taste good and that **instinctively feel right** works a lot better than trying to manage it with *engineered nutrition pretending to be smarter than nature*.

SERVINGS› 12–15
TIME› 20 minutes + time
to cook rice

BAKED RICE BALLS

When we were serving up portables at Ironman Hawaii, we didn't have our trailer along, so we set up shop in a pizza joint. We served up Honey Banana and Ham & Pineapple rice balls because we wanted to give the triathletes a smaller bite. Pick your flavor combination, pulse in a food processor, and press a fistful of sticky rice into whatever shape you like.

DATE & ALMOND

Add ¼ cup almond flour if mixture is too wet.

2 cups uncooked sticky rice
3 cups water

½ cup pitted dates
½ cup sliced almonds
1 tablespoon brown sugar
1 teaspoon ground cinnamon
1½ teaspoons coarse salt

You can substitute ¼ cup shredded unsweetened coconut for the brown sugar.

LEMON RICOTTA

2 cups uncooked sticky rice
3 cups water

½ cup ricotta cheese
1 egg, lightly beaten
2 tablespoons raw sugar
juice of 1 lemon
1½ teaspoons lemon zest

You don't need a food processor to make this variety—just whisk the ingredients together in a large bowl.

HONEY BANANA

2 cups uncooked sticky rice
3 cups water

1 ripe medium banana
1 tablespoon walnuts
1 tablespoon honey

PEACHES & COCONUT CREAM

2 cups uncooked sticky rice
3 cups water

½ cup peeled peaches (fresh or canned)
½ cup canned coconut milk
¼ teaspoon vanilla extract
½ teaspoon coarse salt
1 teaspoon coarse cane sugar

See instructions for making Baked Rice Balls, page 215.

Nutrition facts for recipes can be found in Appendix A, and nutrition for optional additions can be found in Appendix B.

Date &
Almond

Lemon
Ricotta

Ham &
Pineapple

TIP Make a quick batch
of BAKED RICE BALLS
using 2–3 cups of warm
rice left over from dinner.

Sweet Potato
& Bacon

HAM & PINEAPPLE

2 cups uncooked sticky rice

3 cups water

¼ cup chopped cooked ham `COOKED`

¼ cup minced fresh pineapple

2 teaspoons brown sugar

1 teaspoon low-sodium soy sauce

You can use canned pineapple,
thoroughly drained.

PER SERVING› Energy 260 cal, **Fat** 1 g, **Sodium** 85 mg, **Carbs** 57 g, **Fiber** 1 g, **Protein** 5 g, **Water** 57%

BARBEQUE CHICKEN

2 cups uncooked sticky rice

3 cups water

¼ cup minced cooked chicken `COOKED`

1 tablespoon barbeque sauce

2 teaspoons apple cider vinegar

1 tablespoon shredded cheddar cheese

1 teaspoon Old Bay Seasoning

Mix in minced crystallized ginger or orange marmalade for a more adventurous flavor.

POTATO & SWEET GINGER

1 cup uncooked sticky rice

1½ cups water

2 small potatoes, peeled, cooked, and mashed (~1½ cups) `COOKED`

1½ teaspoons minced crystallized ginger

1 tablespoon brown sugar

SWEET & SOUR CHICKEN

2 cups uncooked sticky rice

3 cups water

¼ cup minced cooked chicken `COOKED`

4 teaspoons brown sugar

1 teaspoon rice wine vinegar

1 teaspoon low-sodium soy sauce or liquid aminos

CURRY PUMPKIN DATE

2 cups uncooked sticky rice

3 cups water

½ cup cooked mashed pumpkin `COOKED`

2 tablespoons pitted chopped dates

1 tablespoon chopped pecans

2 teaspoons mild curry powder

If you are using canned pumpkin, add one egg, lightly beaten, to bind the ingredients together.

2 teaspoons brown sugar

1 teaspoon coarse salt

See instructions for making Baked Rice Balls, page 215.

Nutrition facts for recipes can be found in Appendix A, and nutrition facts for optional additions can be found in Appendix B.

SPICY BLACK BEAN

2 cups uncooked sticky rice

3 cups water

½ cup canned black beans, drained and mashed

1 tablespoon Mexican Spice Mix (see recipe, below)

2 teaspoons brown sugar

1 tablespoon brown rice flour

SWEET POTATO & BACON

1 cup uncooked sticky rice

1½ cups water

1 sweet potato, peeled, cooked, and mashed (~1½ cups) COOKED

¼ cup cooked bacon COOKED

½ teaspoon olive oil

1 teaspoon brown sugar

1 teaspoon ground cumin or Mexican Spice Mix (see recipe, below)

sprinkle of coarse salt

MEXICAN SPICE MIX

3 tablespoons ground dark red chili powder

2 teaspoons ground cumin

2 teaspoons ground cinnamon

OPTIONAL ADDITIONS

1 teaspoon ground oregano

1 teaspoon ground black pepper

½ teaspoon onion powder

¼ teaspoon garlic powder

Mix together well.

Store in a small, airtight container. Keeps for several months.

PER SERVING

Spicy Black Bean › Energy 269 cal, Fat 1 g, Sodium 48 mg, Carbs 59 g, Fiber 3 g, Protein 6 g, Water 57%
Sweet Potato & Bacon › Energy 145 cal, Fat 2 g, Sodium 123 mg, Carbs 28 g, Fiber 1 g, Protein 4 g, Water 59%

TO MAKE BAKED RICE BALLS

Combine the water and rice in a rice cooker with a dash of salt and let cook.

While the rice is cooking, place remaining ingredients in a food processor and pulse a few times to get a uniform "minced" finish. (Alternatively, mince the ingredients and stir together in a medium bowl.)

Heat oven to 350 degrees. Lightly coat a baking sheet with nonstick cooking spray or line with parchment paper. When the rice has finished cooking, mix it with the remaining ingredients and stir thoroughly.

Line a small bowl or shape with plastic wrap and press rice mixture into shape. Remove rice ball from plastic wrap and place on baking sheet. (See How to Shape Baked Rice Balls, page 216.) Repeat with remaining rice mixture.

Bake for 10–15 minutes.

Let cool before wrapping.

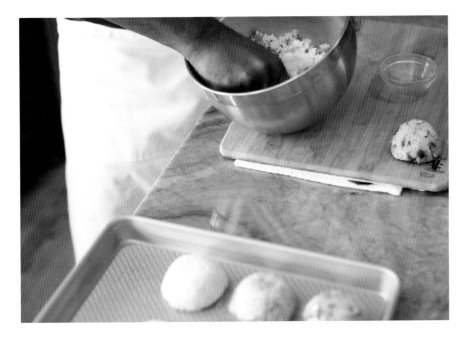

TIP If you like the lighter **TEXTURE** of baked rice balls, try making your favorite rice cake into a ball.

HOW TO SHAPE BAKED RICE BALLS

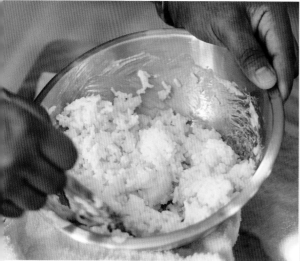

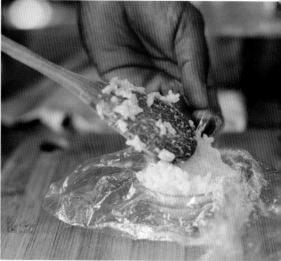

⭐1 Prepare your favorite flavor of baked rice balls.

⭐2 Line a small bowl or shape with plastic wrap and fill with a heaping spoonful of the rice mixture.

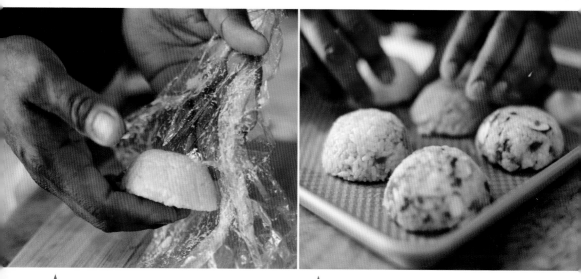

⭐5 Gently remove the rice ball from the wrap.

⭐6 Place the rice ball on the baking sheet and repeat steps 2–5.

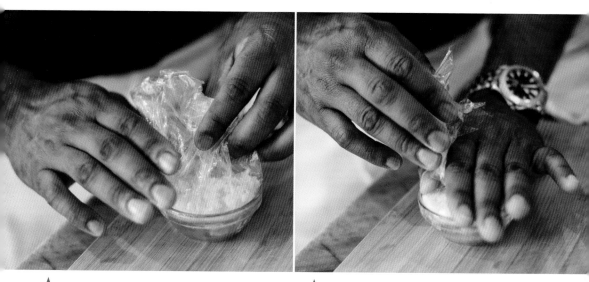

★ Gather up the excess plastic wrap.

★ Firmly press the rice mixture into the shape.

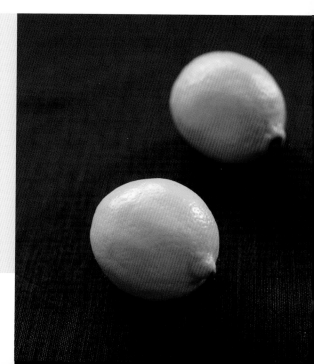

TIP WHEN YOU ARE TRAVELING, A SQUEEZE OF FRESH LEMON BRIGHTENS ANY DISH, WHETHER SWEET OR SAVORY.

"When I'm riding 5 hours or longer, I have tried sushi rice with egg as well as sushi rice with some crunchy peanut butter and honey— it's a winner. Homemade but simple seems to get me through."

TIM DON

ITU WORLD CHAMPION ★ 3-TIME OLYMPIAN ★ 5-TIME BRITISH TRIATHLON CHAMPION

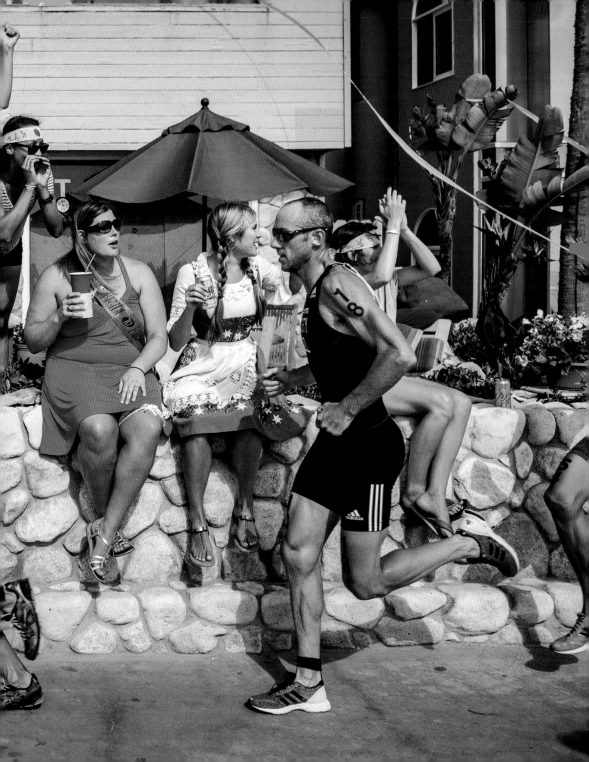

SERVINGS› 12
TIME› 15 minutes prep + time
to cook rice or pasta

STICKY BITES

Most athletes are used to eating gels or energy blocks. A sticky bite uses everyday ingredients to deliver that sweet kick in a more palatable way. The moisture in the carbs (rice, pasta, bread, or oats) allows the body to more quickly digest the nutrition.

CHERRY CHOCOLATE

1 cup uncooked sticky rice

1½ cups water

2 tablespoons cream cheese

2 tablespoons cherry preserves
(or your favorite jam)

¼ teaspoon vanilla extract

FOLD IN

¼ cup bittersweet chocolate chips

TOP WITH

½ teaspoon coarse salt

BLUEBERRY COCONUT

4 ounces uncooked orzo
or other small pasta

2 tablespoons cream cheese

2 tablespoons plain Greek yogurt

2 tablespoons unsweetened
shredded coconut

1½ teaspoons raw sugar

¼ teaspoon vanilla extract

FOLD IN

¼ cup fresh blueberries

TOP WITH

raw sugar + coarse salt

TO MAKE STICKY BITES

Cook the rice or pasta and let cool to the touch. ←

To keep your bites sticky, cook pasta until al dente and don't add oil after draining the water.

In a small food processor, combine the rice or pasta and the sticky and wet ingredients. Pulse until you have a coarse, sticky mixture. Transfer to a medium bowl.

Fold in chocolate chips or blueberries. Sprinkle with topping. ←

Be careful not to add too much salt here.

Press into an airtight container or wrap up in individual shapes.

See instructions for storing and wrapping sticky bites, page 227.

PER SERVING
Cherry Chocolate› Energy 89 cal, Fat 2 g, Sodium 108 mg, Carbs 17 g, Fiber 0 g, Protein 1 g, Water 63%
Blueberry Coconut› Energy 54 cal, Fat 1 g, Sodium 18 mg, Carbs 8 g, Fiber 0 g, Protein 2 g, Water 42%

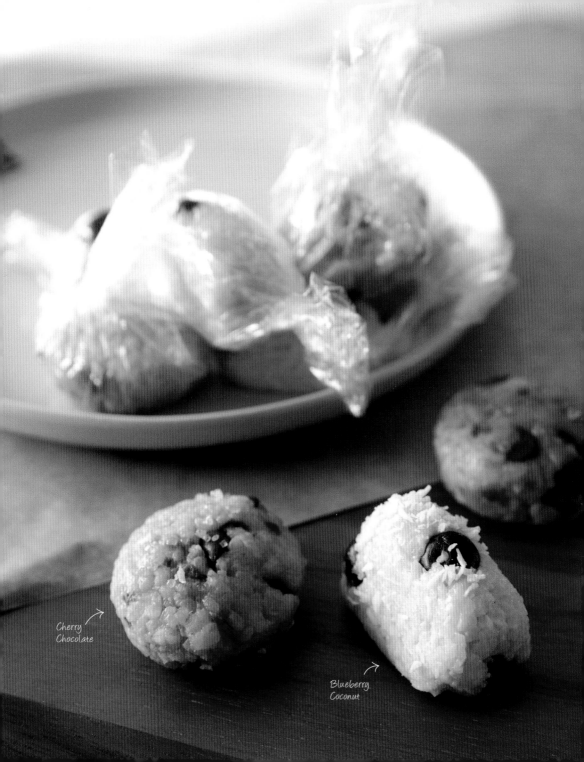

Cherry
Chocolate

Blueberry
Coconut

CARROT CAKE

2 cups cubed gluten-free bread

1 medium carrot (~¼ cup), peeled and grated

2 tablespoons cream cheese

2 tablespoons walnuts

½ teaspoon vanilla extract

1 tablespoon sugar

1 teaspoon cinnamon

dash of salt

If you don't have gluten-free bread, use whatever you have on hand.

Place the bread in a food processor and pulse until you have an even, crumbly consistency.

Combine the remaining ingredients in the food processor. Pulse until you have a sticky mixture that holds together.

Press into an airtight storage container or wrap up individual bites.

See instructions for storing and wrapping sticky bites, page 227.

PER SERVING› **Energy** 55 cal. **Fat** 2 g. **Sodium** 93 mg. **Carbs** 7 g. **Fiber** 0 g. **Protein** 1 g. **Water** 54%

BITTER CHOCOLATE & SEA SALT

1 cup uncooked sticky rice

½ cup uncooked rolled oats

2 cups water

1 tablespoon brown sugar

2 tablespoons bittersweet chocolate (chips or shaved)

¼ teaspoon vanilla extract

dash of sea salt

TOP WITH

2 tablespoons shaved bittersweet chocolate

½ teaspoon sea salt

Combine oats, rice, and water with a dash of salt in a rice cooker and cook. Let cool to the touch.

In a medium bowl, combine the cooked rice and oats with the remaining ingredients. Stir to incorporate the flavor throughout the sticky mixture.

Press into an airtight storage container or shape as individual bites. Sprinkle with chocolate and salt.

See instructions for storing and wrapping sticky bites, page 227.

Be careful not to add too much salt here.

TIP OATS do not contain gluten, but they are often processed in plants where wheat products are made.

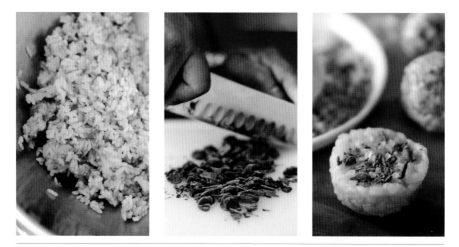

PER SERVING› Energy 101 cal, **Fat** 1 g, **Sodium** 197 mg, **Carbs** 20 g, **Fiber** 1 g, **Protein** 2 g, **Water** 64%

SESAME HONEY & COCONUT

1 cup uncooked sticky rice

1½ cups water

2 tablespoons sesame seeds

2 tablespoons unsweetened
shredded coconut

1 tablespoon honey

¼ teaspoon vanilla extract

½ teaspoon salt

Combine the rice, water, and a dash of salt in a rice cooker and cook. Let cool to the touch.

In a dry sauté pan over medium heat, lightly toast the sesame seeds and shredded coconut until golden. Set aside half of the mixture for topping.

In a food processor, combine the cooked rice with the remaining ingredients. Pulse a few times until you have a coarse, sticky mixture.

Top with the remaining toasted sesame seed and coconut mixutre.

See instructions for storing and wrapping sticky bites, page 227.

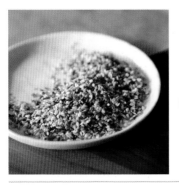

TIP Enhance the flavor of nuts, seeds, or coconut by **TOASTING** in a dry pan before adding to your recipe. Skip this step when you are short on time.

PER SERVING› Energy 77 cal, **Fat** 1 g, **Sodium** 99 mg, **Carbs** 15 g, **Fiber** 1 g, **Protein** 1 g, **Water** 64%

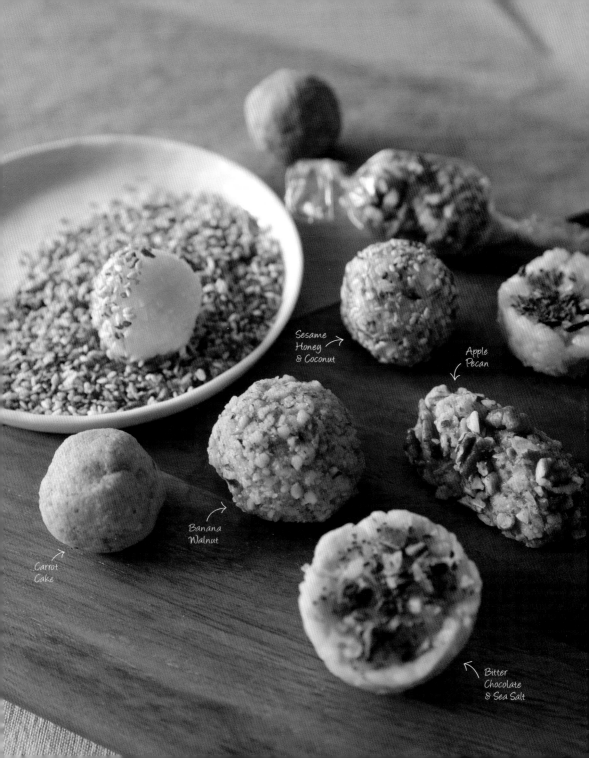

Sesame
Honey
& Coconut

Apple
Pecan

Banana
Walnut

Carrot
Cake

Bitter
Chocolate
& Sea Salt

APPLE PECAN

1½ cups water

1 cup uncooked rolled oats

¼ teaspoon vanilla extract

¼ cup coarsely chopped apple

2 tablespoons pecans

1 tablespoon brown sugar

1 teaspoon ground cinnamon

dash of salt

BANANA WALNUT

1½ cups water

1 cup uncooked rolled oats

¼ teaspoon vanilla extract

1 medium banana

2 slices gluten-free bread

2 tablespoons walnuts

1 tablespoon brown sugar

dash of salt

TO MAKE STICKY BITES

In a small saucepan bring water to a boil with a dash of salt. Add the oats, and cook over medium-high heat, stirring frequently. Cook for 5 minutes or until most of the water has been absorbed. Add the vanilla, remove from heat, and set aside.

Place the remaining ingredients in a small food processor and pulse a few times to combine. Transfer to a medium bowl and fold in the cooked oats.

Press into a small baking pan or individual shapes and top with additional chopped nuts or coarse salt.

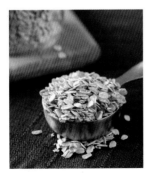

TIP When using **OATS** in sticky bites, for the best texture fold them in after the other ingredients have been pulsed in the food processor.

PER SERVING
Apple Pecan› Energy 66 cal, **Fat** 2 g, **Sodium** 10 mg, **Carbs** 11 g, **Fiber** 2 g, **Protein** 2 g, **Water** 69%
Banana Walnut› Energy 83 cal, **Fat** 2 g, **Sodium** 35 mg, **Carbs** 14 g, **Fiber** 2 g, **Protein** 3 g, **Water** 65%

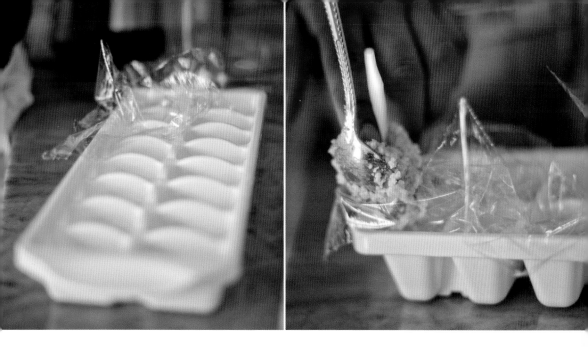

STORING & WRAPPING STICKY BITES

Sticky bites can be stored in the refrigerator in an airtight container or individually wrapped. **STORE**› Press the sticky mixture into a shallow airtight container and top with plastic wrap. Simply cut and wrap bites as you need them. **WRAP**› Place a heaping tablespoon of the sticky mixture on a small piece of plastic wrap. Press into a shape like an ice cube or spoon. Roll plastic wrap lengthwise and then twist the ends like a hard candy wrapper.

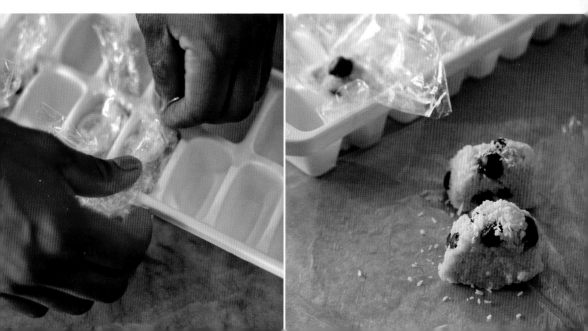

IDLI is a combination of hulled black lentils and soaked rice that are ground together and, when prepared traditionally, left to ferment overnight. The fermentation gives the finished cakes a light, savory finish that goes great with spicy sauces as well as jams and honey.

IDLI

This is a type of steamed rice cake popular in southern India. Growing up, Biju would eat these most every day for breakfast or as a snack, so he's delighted to see idli popping up on mainstream menus across the country. Traditionally, idli is made in a steamer pan with oval-shaped forms. We've simplified the method to use a mix available at most Indian markets and whatever small, shallow cups or bowls you have on hand.

1 cup instant idli mix

1–1½ cups cold water

See the instructions on the idli mix packaging for a more precise water measurement.

In a small bowl, combine the idli mix with 1 cup of cold water. If needed, gradually add more water until you have a thick mixture that is slightly lumpy or gritty. Set aside for 10 minutes.

Meanwhile, fill a rice cooker or a steamer with approximately 2 inches of water and bring to a slow, rolling boil over medium-high heat.

Lightly coat small cups or bowls with nonstick cooking spray. When the idli mix is finished resting, fill the cups no more than ½ full. Use tongs to place the cups in the steamer tray.

Espresso cups work well.

Cover and steam for approximately 10 minutes, or until the mixture becomes firm. Remove from heat.

Let cool to the touch before flipping each bowl or cup over in your hand to remove the idli. Wrap and pack for your next ride.

TIP There are a number of batters you can prepare with this method: Cream of Wheat, quick polenta, Cream of Rice. Simply mix with equal parts water, and **STEAM** until firm.

PER SERVING› Energy 105 cal, **Fat** 0 g, **Sodium** 332 mg, **Carbs** 21 g, **Fiber** 0 g, **Protein** 3 g, **Water** 57%

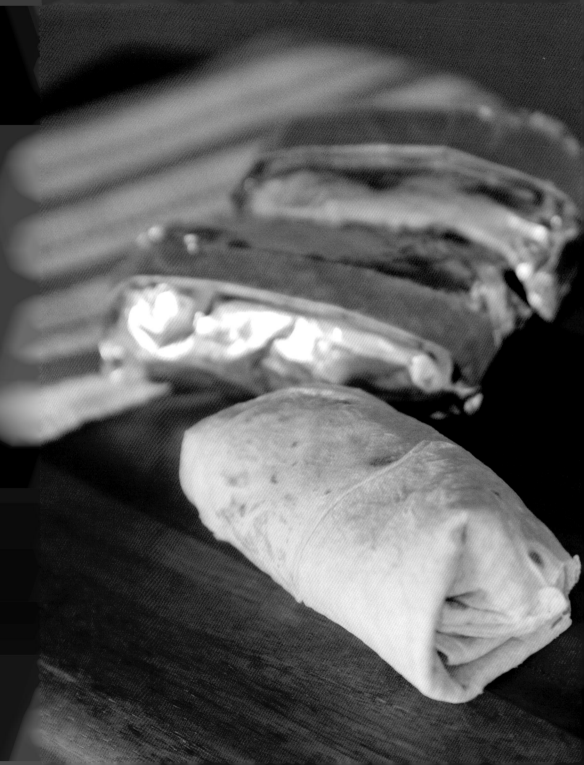

TAKE & MAKE

We often hear from athletes who cook on the road just like us. They pack up a portable kitchen with a hot plate, rice cooker, and some bowls or pans, and they can turn out any number of items from virtually anywhere. If that sounds daunting, start out with something a little more straightforward. With a little prep work, you can have Biju's oatmeal mix or Liège waffle dough packed and ready. Our other Take & Make items are simple ideas on how to put together food that is readily available everywhere.

V VEGETARIAN   **G** GLUTEN-FREE

PORTABLE OATMEAL

You can take any hearty granola and pour hot milk over it to have "instant" oatmeal when you are on the road. We've stayed pretty true to our original oatmeal since it is a pre-race favorite.

½ cup apple juice or
pineapple juice

1 ripe banana, mashed

1 cup honey or agave nectar

1 cup sliced almonds (4 ounces)

1 teaspoon ground cinnamon

½ teaspoon coarse salt

4 cups rolled oats (16 ounces)

1 cup raisins or
chopped dried fruit

OPTIONAL ADDITIONS

1 teaspoon vanilla extract

¼ teaspoon ground nutmeg

1 cup unsalted cashews
(4 ounces)

*You can substitute ½ cup
applesauce for the banana.*

Heat oven to 350 degrees. Lightly coat a 13" × 18" (half sheet) baking pan with cooking spray or line with parchment paper.

Add vanilla and nutmeg here if using.

Place the juice, banana, and honey in a blender or small food processor and puree into a smooth mixture. Transfer to a large bowl.

Stir in the almonds, cinnamon, salt, and oats and let soak for about 10 minutes.

Add cashews here if using.

Spread evenly onto the baking sheet and bake on the center rack of the oven for 20 minutes.

Stir mixture thoroughly and cook for another 20 minutes.

Stir mixture a final time, add dried fruit, and cook for an additional 10 minutes or until the oats are golden. Remove from oven while granola is still a bit undercooked.

Let cool, then store in an airtight container or portion into ziplock bags. Makes about 6 cups.

TAKE & MAKE

Heat your favorite milk and pour over an equal amount of the granola. Cover and let rest for a few minutes. The granola will become creamy oatmeal as it soaks up the warm milk.

PER SERVING› **Energy** 400 cal, **Fat** 9 g, **Sodium** 98 mg, **Carbs** 75 g, **Fiber** 7 g, **Protein** 11 g, **Water** 24%
Nutrition facts for optional additions can be found in Appendix B.

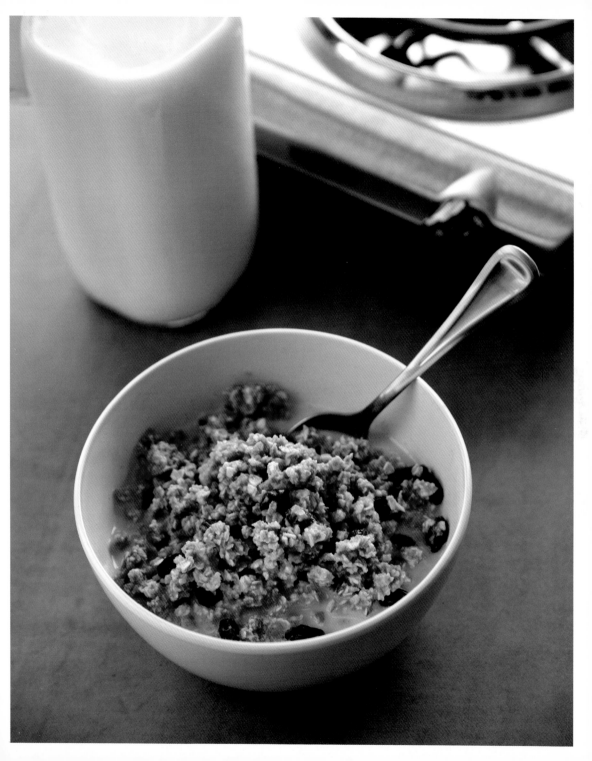

TOASTED NUT MIX

We changed up our basic recipe from *The Feed Zone Cookbook* to be more affordable and accessible. Use whatever nuts you have on hand in the ratios provided.

1 cup chopped pecans

1 cup slivered almonds

1 cup unsweetened shredded coconut

½ cup chopped dates or other dried fruit

Heat oven to 350 degrees.

Combine the nuts, shredded coconut, and dates or dried fruit on a baking sheet.

Bake for about 12–15 minutes, or until coconut begins to toast.

Let cool and store in an airtight container.

TIP› Toasted Nut Mix is a **BRILLIANT SNACK** when you are on the road.

PER SERVING› Energy 132 cal, Fat 10 g, Sodium 4 mg, Carbs 12 g, Fiber 3 g, Protein 2 g, Water 11%

★★★

"My gold medal ride in London was fueled by Biju's Oatmeal. I told Allen to change the name to Gold Medal Oatmeal. It took a team to win— I left my nutrition to the experts and they left the ride to me."

KRISTIN ARMSTRONG
2-TIME OLYMPIC GOLD MEDALIST, TIME TRIAL
2-TIME UCI WORLD CHAMPION, TIME TRIAL

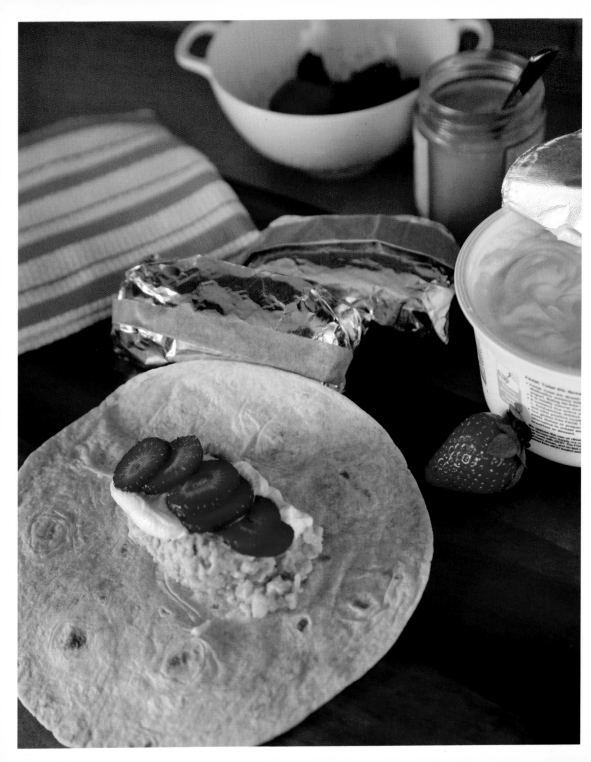

SWEET BREAKFAST BURRITO

This is a sweet new twist on the classic breakfast burrito. It passes the no-mess test because as the oatmeal cools, the oats will continue to absorb any excess moisture.

2 flour tortillas (8-inch)

COOKED 1 cup cooked oatmeal

¼ cup fresh berries

2 tablespoons plain Greek yogurt

2 tablespoons Toasted Nut Mix (see page 234)

drizzle of honey (optional)

Divide the oatmeal between the two tortillas. Top with your favorite berries, a dollop of yogurt, and a small handful of Toasted Nut Mix.

Tuck in the short edges and tightly roll the burrito lengthwise.

Wrap in paper foil or plastic wrap. Store in the refrigerator for up to 48 hours.

TO MAKE FRESH OATMEAL

In a medium saucepan, bring **1 cup of water** with a dash of salt to a low boil. ★ Add **1 cup old-fashioned rolled oats** and cook, stirring frequently, about 5 minutes. ★ Add **½ cup milk** and return to a low boil. (Add more milk to reach a thick consistency.) ★ Flavor with **1 tablespoon brown sugar** and **1 tablespoon molasses**. Remove the pan from the heat. ★ Let rest 10–15 minutes.

Note› *This makes almost 2 cups of cooked oatmeal, so there's enough to enjoy a bowlful before you roll up burritos or save some for your next day's batch.*

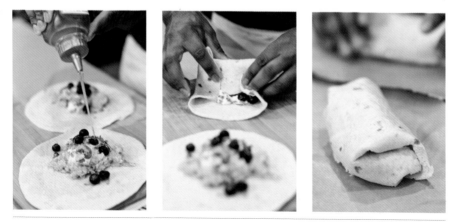

PER SERVING› Energy 319 cal, **Fat** 10 g, **Sodium** 261 mg, **Carbs** 51 g, **Fiber** 4 g, **Protein** 10 g, **Water** 62%

TIP SURPRISINGLY ENOUGH, MOST HOTELS HAVE A **WAFFLE IRON** AS PART OF THEIR CONTINENTAL BREAKFAST SETUP. JAM YOUR DOUGH IN THERE WHEN NO ONE'S LOOKING.

LIÈGE WAFFLES

If you have ever been to Europe to watch a bike race, you have probably enjoyed one of these waffles. This recipe has been simplified somewhat, but plan to let the dough rest in the fridge overnight for light, flavorful waffles.

¾ cup milk, warmed

1 tablespoon active dry yeast

1 tablespoon cane sugar

3 cups flour

3 large eggs

1 tablespoon maple syrup or honey

½ cup melted butter

2 teaspoons vanilla extract

½ teaspoon salt

small bowl of pearled sugar

You can use coarse sugar in place of pearled sugar.

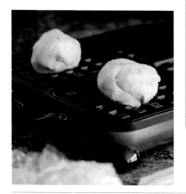

Place milk, yeast, cane sugar, and 1 cup of flour in a bowl and mix into a soft dough using an electric mixer. Let dough rest for about 15 minutes.

In a bowl, whisk together eggs, maple syrup or honey, butter, and vanilla. Add egg mixture to dough along with the remaining flour and salt. Mix well into a soft sticky dough. Cover and let rise in a warm place for 1 hour.

Punch down the dough and scrape it from the sides of the bowl. Loosely cover with plastic wrap and let rest in fridge overnight.

Divide dough into 12 portions, shape each into a small ball, and roll in pearled sugar. Wrap individually in plastic wrap and store in an airtight container or ziplock bag.

Once individually wrapped, you can freeze the dough.

TAKE & MAKE

Heat the waffle iron. Press the dough onto the iron and cook until color is golden and waffle feels crisp to the touch.

TO MAKE INDULGENT DESSERT WAFFLES

Add to the recipe 2 tablespoons sugar, 1 egg yolk, ½ cup of melted butter, and 1 teaspoon of baking powder. Use an extra ½ cup flour, or just enough to keep the dough a bit sticky.

PER SERVING› Energy 228 cal, **Fat** 10 g, **Sodium** 126 mg, **Carbs** 29 g, **Fiber** 1 g, **Protein** 6 g, **Water** 39%

ALLEN'S MOCHIKO KRISPIES

Allen set out to make a bar that would meet all of his standards for carbohydrates and moisture content and be no-fuss enough to make in a hotel in just minutes. These bars use mochi flour, a sweet rice flour available in Asian markets, as a substitute for the traditional marshmallows.

½ cup almond milk

½ cup mochi flour

2 tablespoons butter

2 tablespoons sugar

2 cups brown rice crisp cereal

½ cup chocolate chips (optional)

Combine the milk, mochi flour, butter, and sugar in a medium microwave-safe bowl. Cook in the microwave on high for 1 minute.

Stir, then return to microwave for another 1½–2 minutes.

Add chocolate chips here if using.

Add the cereal and stir to fully incorporate.

Spread the mixture into a greased baking pan or onto wax paper.

Let cool for at least 15 minutes before cutting and wrapping.

TIP MOCHI FLOUR is the magical ingredient here. All-purpose flour is not a suitable substitution. Rice

PER SERVING› Energy 210 cal, Fat 6 g, Sodium 100 mg, Carbs 36 g, Fiber 0 g, Protein 3 g, Water 40%
(with chocolate)› Energy 287 cal, Fat 11 g, Sodium 103 mg, Carbs 44 g, Fiber 1 g, Protein 3 g, Water 34%

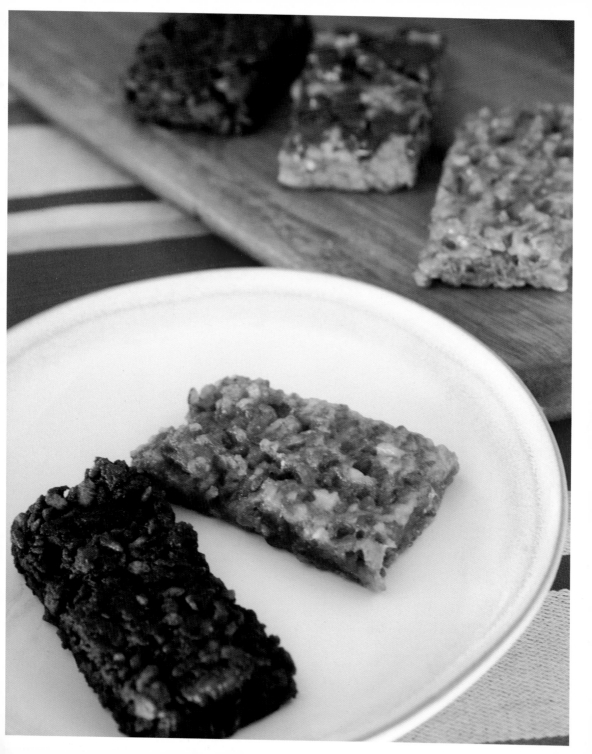

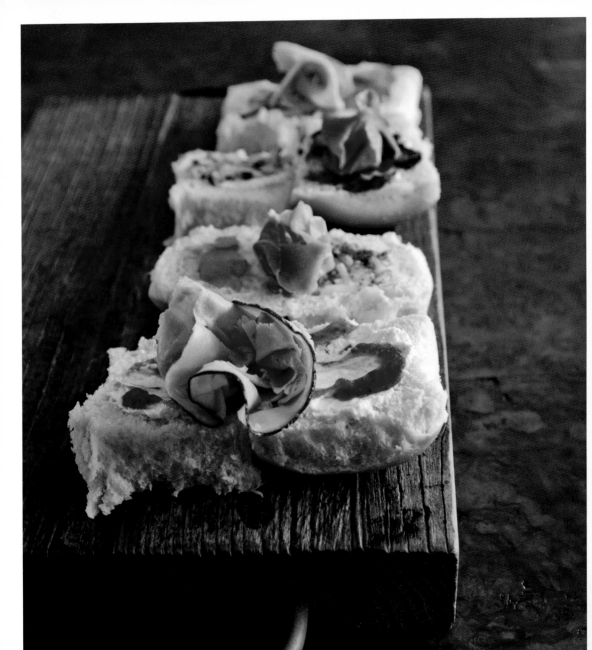

TIP SOFT DINNER ROLLS AND SMALL BREADS WORK BEST. RUSTIC OR CRUSTY BREADS ARE MESSY AND TOO DIFFICULT TO EAT IN ONE OR TWO BITES.

THE RIDE "PANINI"

The riders refer to any variety of small, easy-to-eat sandwiches as paninis. The classic combination is a sliver of meat, cheese, and some jam. Mix and match your favorite combinations of fully cooked meats or other proteins and flavors and top with chopped pickles or nuts. Here are some ideas to get you started.

prosciutto + cream cheese + raspberry jam

peanut butter + grape jam + chopped nuts

smoked turkey + Swiss cheese + spreadable honey

mild smoked chorizo, chopped + mashed avocado

chopped bacon + mashed avocado + smoked salmon bits

pumpkin butter + cream cheese + pecan pieces

ham + cream cheese + raspberry jam + caramelized onions

peanut butter + minced dates + banana slices

Nutella + cream cheese + spreadable honey

smoked chicken + brie + ripe banana

almond butter + chopped dried figs + toasted almond pieces

roast beef + feta + pickle relish

Do pickles really stop cramping? See page 245.

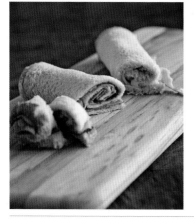

ROLLED SANDWICHES

Again, this is all about easy bites. Roll out fresh, soft bread slices for a compact, no-mess portable.

Use a rolling pin or wine bottle to roll out a slice of bread until it is thin and pliable.

Add sandwich fillings, taking care to spread them evenly.

Roll it up and wrap tightly as bites or rolls.

Nutrition facts for optional additions can be found in Appendix B.

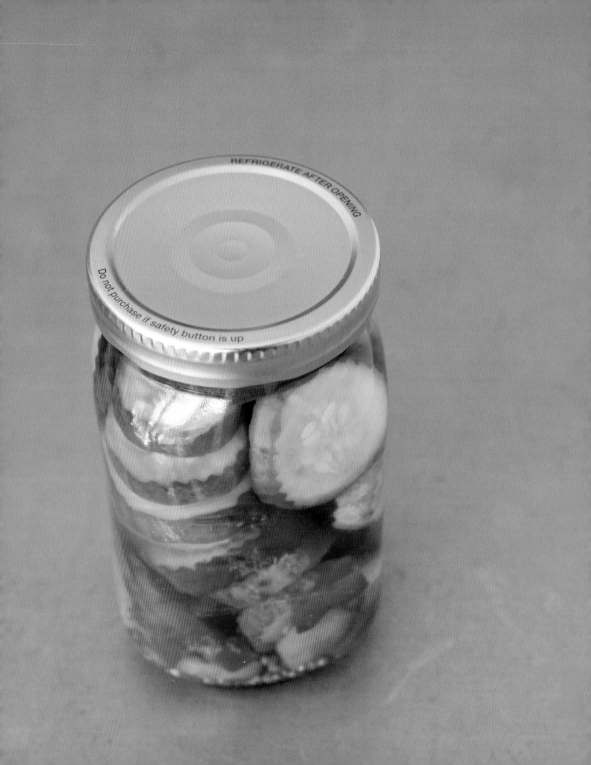

For years athletic trainers have used PICKLE JUICE as a remedy for exercise-associated muscle cramps, claiming that a Dixie cup full of the salty and acidic brine can stop a cramp in less than a minute. Cramps can be caused by muscle fatigue as well as severe dehydration and sodium loss, all of which can increase the risk for errant reflexes, which initiate involuntary neural signals that are at the center of all cramps. So drinking something really salty might help counter one potential cramping mechanism. Testing this idea, Kevin Miller at North Dakota State University along with colleagues at Brigham Young University developed a model for creating electrically induced muscle cramps in dehydrated subjects to see if drinking pickle juice really worked.

Long story short, pickle juice relieved the cramping. But it happened more quickly than the body could deliver the extra salt or the small amount of water. For that reason, the researchers suggested that the cramping was stopped because of an oropha-ryngeal reflex that inhibited the neural signals causing the cramp. Essentially, the pickle juice tickled the subject's mid-throat, sending a neural signal that overpowered the neural signal causing the cramp—a lightning bolt of sourness that created an electrical storm through the body, short-circuiting the short circuit that caused the cramp.

When I mentioned this to Chef Biju, he immediately got it, blurting out "Like ume plum vinegar!" as he shuddered in sour shock. Chef Biju claims that this type of vinegar, made from sea salt and the pickling brine of the umeboshi plum, will induce a throat tickle, back of tongue drool, and sour patch headshake that rivals all sour tickle drool shakes. While I've never personally used either pickle juice or ume plum vinegar to stop cramps, the rationale is there for any of us to try it.

But until then, you can prevent cramps by getting plenty of water and electrolytes before and during exercise and making sure you have adequate fuel and training under your legs so you won't have to summon the strength to knock someone over for their pickle juice in the middle of a workout or race.

★ ★ ★

"I travel extensively in many different countries, so I am always in search of a dependable solution to my portable energy food needs. Simple, nutritious ingredients and easy preparation are a winning combination when it comes to keeping yourself healthy on the road."

CARLO TRAVERSI
2-TIME SPORT CLIMBING NATIONAL CHAMPION
5-TIME USA CLIMBING NATIONAL TEAM

This book is an acknowledgment that we can't outsmart nature. ★ It's an effort to *keep things simple, share ideas*, and further a discussion that we know has improved the **health and performance** of the athletes and friends we've cooked for.

APPENDIXES

APPENDIX A
NUTRITION FACTS FOR RECIPES

What follows are the nutrition totals for each recipe, organized by section. This is helpful because you can quickly calculate the nutrition facts for a given recipe if you decide to adjust the portions.

RICE CAKES

RECIPE	ENERGY (CAL)	FAT (G)	SODIUM (MG)	CARB (G)	FIBER (G)	PROTEIN (G)	WATER (%)
Blueberry & Chocolate Coconut Rice Cakes	3,733	94	2,903	668	28	53	65
Cinnamon Apple Rice Cakes	2,389	4	2,607	539	13	39	68
The Denver Rice Cake	2,777	51	1,165	471	9	92	71
Masala Chicken Rice Cakes	2,681	35	992	490	11	90	66
PB&J Rice Cakes	4,513	134	1,432	736	27	105	56
Raspberry & Mint Rice Cakes	2,637	5	152	598	25	42	68
Red Lentil Rice Cakes	2,253	17	1,656	443	31	82	67
Spiced Beef & Onion Rice Cakes	2,966	15	896	606	10	88	65
Swiss Rice Cakes	2,662	71	1,140	424	18	72	68

BAKED EGGS

RECIPE	ENERGY (CAL)	FAT (G)	SODIUM (MG)	CARB (G)	FIBER (G)	PROTEIN (G)	WATER (%)
Baked Eggs	481	34	1,068	3	0	41	63
Crispy Rice Omelet	795	48	1,608	41	2	48	46
Mushroom & Swiss Frittata	1,042	52	1,753	91	7	54	65
Potato & Leek Frittata	481	19	1,336	39	3	39	65
Rice Soufflé	828	39	2,011	43	2	75	60
Spinach & Zucchini Frittata	625	38	820	37	5	37	67

TWO-BITE PIES

RECIPE	ENERGY (CAL)	FAT (G)	SODIUM (MG)	CARB (G)	FIBER (G)	PROTEIN (G)	WATER (%)
Gluten-Free Pie Crust	1,908	78	3,499	253	11	52	12
Quick Crust	563	36	490	36	2	6	12
Traditional Pie Crust	2,442	125	1,192	287	11	40	18
Warm Dough	1,493	8	287	305	12	41	19
Apple filling	548	0	2,357	141	6	1	46
Banana Walnut filling	491	20	7	81	10	8	54
Beef & Sweet Potato filling	945	29	4,502	115	8	54	61
Black Bean & Peanut Molé filling	1,264	56	2,625	156	31	46	22
Blueberry filling	729	21	239	134	5	5	45
Curry Potato & Chicken filling	628	24	1,925	83	7	26	65
Golden Beet & Chicken Pot Pie filling	627	34	5,301	39	6	44	67
Molé Sauce	1,286	90	313	98	22	44	54
Strawberries & Cream filling	324	9	68	55	7	9	72

BAKED CAKES & COOKIES

RECIPE	ENERGY (CAL)	FAT (G)	SODIUM (MG)	CARB (G)	FIBER (G)	PROTEIN (G)	WATER (%)
Chocolate Cakes	1,280	67	1,301	144	12	30	30
Chocolate Chip Cookies	1,090	32	1,391	181	12	21	43
Crispy Grits	1,443	26	2,252	257	6	42	64
French Toast Cakes	825	32	1,392	95	6	40	63
Mushroom & Thyme Bread Cake	1,191	45	4,101	142	10	59	62
Nut Butter Cookies	1,120	46	1,009	183	13	25	31
Sausage & Potato Cakes	1,283	48	4,826	160	10	54	53
Snickerdoodle Cookies	1,005	22	762	181	10	20	33
Spiced Pumpkin Cakes	1,295	70	2,754	115	9	53	45
Spinach & Red Pepper Polenta Cakes	1,339	16	3,472	258	6	33	71
Sweet Cream Grits	1,359	17	163	258	5	36	65

GRIDDLE CAKES, PANCAKES, & WAFFLES

RECIPE	ENERGY (CAL)	FAT (G)	SODIUM (MG)	CARB (G)	FIBER (G)	PROTEIN (G)	WATER (%)
Banana Waffles	897	28	483	138	10	28	43
Beet Juice Waffle Sandwiches	962	34	501	137	3	27	50
Carrot Waffles	893	34	299	119	4	27	41
Cheesy Potato Waffles	920	30	2,266	122	10	41	35
Griddle Cakes	770	7	154	153	6	20	27
Mashed Potato Cakes	498	22	1,395	50	4	25	70
Scallion Pancakes	581	15	1,173	97	4	13	43
Sweet Corn Cakes	1,104	40	380	168	13	24	47
Sweet Potato Cakes	1,037	36	392	157	14	24	56

AHA! PORTABLES

RECIPE	ENERGY (CAL)	FAT (G)	SODIUM (MG)	CARB (G)	FIBER (G)	PROTEIN (G)	WATER (%)
Apple Pecan Sticky Bites	786	21	118	126	20	28	69
Baked Pasta	1,622	59	1,466	171	7	96	39
Banana Walnut Sticky Bites	998	24	420	168	22	34	65
Barbeque Chicken Rice Balls	1,512	5	1,084	321	6	34	58
Basic Dough	1,639	25	2,000	302	13	45	32
Bitter Chocolate & Sea Salt Sticky Bites	1,213	15	2,358	237	13	28	64
Blueberry Coconut Sticky Bites	643	18	210	101	6	20	42
Blueberry Kugel	1,553	43	376	220	11	72	35
Carrot Cake Sticky Bites	662	29	1,110	86	6	16	54
Cherry Chocolate Sticky Bites	1,068	20	1,291	200	5	16	63
Cinnamon Rolls	1,364	58	1,002	190	8	22	25
Curry Pumpkin Date Rice Balls	1,609	8	2,020	349	13	29	58
Date & Almond Rice Balls	2,544	39	3,082	519	30	46	46
Ham & Pineapple Rice Balls	1,560	3	512	342	6	32	57
Honey Banana Rice Balls	1,619	7	35	355	9	28	57
Idli	630	–	1,989	126	–	18	57
Lemon Ricotta Rice Balls	1,795	23	206	342	6	46	58

AHA! PORTABLES *(continued)*

RECIPE	ENERGY (CAL)	FAT (G)	SODIUM (MG)	CARB (G)	FIBER (G)	PROTEIN (G)	WATER (%)
Mexican Spice Mix	116	4	230	26	15	4	9
Peaches & Coconut Cream Rice Balls	1,673	27	977	324	7	29	59
Pizza Rolls	866	16	2,379	153	7	25	35
Potato & Sweet Ginger Rice Balls	984	1	465	223	6	17	57
Sesame Honey & Coconut Sticky Bites	918	15	1,184	178	6	17	64
Spicy Black Bean Rice Balls	1,611	4	286	351	17	35	57
Sweet & Sour Chicken Rice Balls	1,507	3	231	327	6	33	57
Sweet Potato & Bacon Rice Balls	868	11	738	168	6	21	59

TAKE & MAKE

RECIPE	ENERGY (CAL)	FAT (G)	SODIUM (MG)	CARB (G)	FIBER (G)	PROTEIN (G)	WATER (%)
Allen's Mochiko Krispies	841	25	398	143	1	10	40
Liège Waffles	2,731	115	1,510	349	13	71	39
Portable Oatmeal	4,004	88	976	754	71	106	24
Sweet Breakfast Burrito	638	21	521	101	8	20	62
Toasted Nut Mix	3,174	229	86	287	63	55	11

* Water % adjusted to account for moisture loss during baking or cooking when applicable.

APPENDIX B
NUTRITION FACTS FOR ADDITIONS & ALTERNATIVES

CARBS

INGREDIENT	ENERGY (CAL)	FAT (G)	SODIUM (MG)	CARB (G)	FIBER (G)	PROTEIN (G)	WATER (%)
BREAD› 1 SLICE							
Bread, gluten-free	70	2	150	11	1	2	37
Bread, whole-wheat	69	1	132	12	2	4	39
Bread, buttermilk	60	1	85	11	–	2	38
Bread, potato	90	1	150	18	1	3	35
Bread› 1 dinner roll	76	2	95	13	1	2	37
Tortilla, 8" flour	146	3	249	25	–	4	33
Tortilla, 8" whole wheat	130	2	330	26	3	4	33
GRAINS› 1 CUP COOKED							
Grits	143	–	5	31	1	3	86
Lentils	230	1	4	40	16	18	70
Oats, old-fashioned rolled	166	4	9	32	4	6	84
Polenta	146	1	3	32	2	3	86
Quinoa	222	4	13	39	5	8	71
FLOURS› 1 CUP							
All-purpose flour	455	1	2	95	3	13	12
Potato flour	571	1	88	133	9	11	6
Rice flour	578	2	–	127	4	9	12
Rice flour, brown	574	4	13	121	7	11	12
PASTA› 1 CUP COOKED							
Angel hair	184	2	120	34	2	8	73
Orzo	200	1	–	42	2	7	72

CARBS *(continued)*

INGREDIENT	ENERGY (CAL)	FAT (G)	SODIUM (MG)	CARB (G)	FIBER (G)	PROTEIN (G)	WATER (%)
RICE> 1 CUP COOKED							
Basmati	220	3	15	44	1	6	77
Brown	218	2	2	46	4	5	73
Jasmine	280	4	18	53	2	6	67
Sticky/calrose (white, medium-grain)	242	–	–	53	1	4	69

FRUITS

INGREDIENT	ENERGY (CAL)	FAT (G)	SODIUM (MG)	CARB (G)	FIBER (G)	PROTEIN (G)	WATER (%)
BERRIES> ½ CUP							
Blackberries	31	1	1	7	4	1	88
Blueberries	42	–	1	11	2	1	85
Raspberries	32	1	1	8	4	1	85
Strawberries	25	–	1	6	2	1	91
DRIED FRUIT> ¼ CUP							
Coconut, unsweetened shredded> 1 tbsp.	33	3	2	1	1	–	3
Cranberries	86	–	1	23	2	–	16
Currants	79	–	2	21	2	1	19
Dates> 1 tbsp.	66	–	–	18	2	–	21
Figs, chopped> 1 tbsp.	21	–	1	5	1	–	31
Raisins	109	–	4	29	1	1	14
FRESH FRUIT							
Avocado> 1 tbsp.	23	2	1	1	1	–	71
Banana> 1 tbsp.	13	–	–	3	–	–	71
Lemon> 1 tbsp. juice	4	–	–	2	–	–	90
Lime> 1 tbsp. juice	4	–	–	2	–	–	90
Peach> 1 medium	59	–	–	15	2	1	89
Pineapple> ½ cup	41	–	1	11	1	1	86

VEGETABLES

INGREDIENT	ENERGY (CAL)	FAT (G)	SODIUM (MG)	CARB (G)	FIBER (G)	PROTEIN (G)	WATER (%)
Beets› ½ cup	37	–	65	8	2	1	87
Bell pepper› ½ cup	9	–	2	2	1	1	89
Carrot› 1 medium, cooked	25	–	42	6	2	1	89
Jalapeno› 1 tbsp.	2	–	–	1	–	–	86
Mushrooms› ½ cup	8	–	2	1	–	1	91
Ginger, grated› 1 tsp.	2	–	–	–	–	–	80
Onion› 1 tbsp.	4	–	–	1	–	–	89
Potato› 1 medium, cooked	145	–	8	34	2	3	76
Scallions/green onions› 1 tbsp.	1	–	–	–	–	–	92
Spinach› ½ cup	4	–	12	1	1	1	88
Sweet potato› 1 medium	103	–	41	24	4	2	75
Tomato› ½ cup	17	–	5	4	1	1	94
FRESH HERBS› 1 TBSP.							
Basil	1	–	1	–	–	–	96
Cilantro	1	–	1	–	–	–	80
Mint	1	–	1	–	–	–	80
Parsley	1	–	1	–	–	–	87
Tarragon	1	–	1	–	–	–	80
Thyme	1	–	1	–	–	–	80

PROTEIN

INGREDIENT	ENERGY (CAL)	FAT (G)	SODIUM (MG)	CARB (G)	FIBER (G)	PROTEIN (G)	WATER (%)
BEANS› 1 CUP COOKED							
Black	227	1	2	41	15	15	66
Red (adzuki)	219	–	7	40	16	16	67
EGGS› 1 EGG							
Baked	71	5	70	–	–	6	64
Fried	90	7	94	–	–	6	69
Poached	71	5	70	–	–	6	74

PROTEIN *(continued)*

INGREDIENT	ENERGY (CAL)	FAT (G)	SODIUM (MG)	CARB (G)	FIBER (G)	PROTEIN (G)	WATER (%)
MEATS› 0.5 OZ.							
Bacon, cooked› 1 slice	41	3	188	–	–	3	13
Chicken, smoked	23	1	134	–	–	3	69
Chicken sausage› 1 link (3 oz.)	180	12	620	4	–	13	81
Chorizo, cooked	64	5	173	–	–	3	32
Ham, deli sliced	15	–	149	–	–	3	74
Prosciutto	29	2	284	–	–	3	64
Smoked salmon bits	16	1	280	–	–	3	72
Smoked turkey	13	–	168	–	–	3	74
NUT BUTTERS› 1 TBSP.							
Almond butter	101	10	72	3	1	2	1
Nutella	100	6	8	12	1	1	1
Peanut butter	94	8	73	3	1	4	2
NUTS & SEEDS› ¼ CUP (1 oz.)							
Almonds	161	14	–	6	3	6	5
Cashews	155	12	3	9	1	5	5
Peanuts	159	14	5	5	2	7	6
Pecans	193	20	–	4	3	3	4
Pumpkin seeds, dried› 1 tbsp.	38	3	1	1	–	2	7
Sesame seeds, dried› 1 tbsp.	52	4	1	2	1	2	4
Walnuts	183	18	1	4	2	4	4

DAIRY

INGREDIENT	ENERGY (CAL)	FAT (G)	SODIUM (MG)	CARB (G)	FIBER (G)	PROTEIN (G)	WATER (%)
CHEESE› 1 OZ.							
Brie	94	8	176	–	–	6	48
Cheddar	113	9	174	–	–	7	37
Feta	74	6	312	1	–	4	55
Fontina	109	9	224	–	–	7	38

INGREDIENT	ENERGY (CAL)	FAT (G)	SODIUM (MG)	CARB (G)	FIBER (G)	PROTEIN (G)	WATER (%)
CHEESE› 1 OZ. *(continued)*							
Goat	102	8	144	1	–	6	45
Monterey jack	104	8	150	–	–	7	41
Mozzarella	84	6	176	1	–	6	50
Parmesan, grated/shredded› 1 tbsp.	22	1	76	–	–	2	20
Swiss cheese	106	8	54	2	–	8	37
CREAM CHEESE & YOGURT› ½ CUP (4 oz.)							
Cream cheese, low-fat› 1 tbsp.	30	2	70	1	–	1	67
Yogurt, Greek, plain, nonfat	67	–	43	5	–	12	78
Yogurt, Greek, plain, full fat	108	4	40	4	–	12	76
Yogurt, plain, low-fat	77	2	86	1	–	1	85
MILK› ½ CUP							
Dairy, 1%	51	1	54	6	–	4	90
Dairy, 2%	61	3	50	6	–	4	89
Dairy, skim/nonfat	43	–	64	6	–	4	91
Dairy, whole	73	4	49	6	–	4	89
Almond, unsweetened	20	2	90	1	–	1	92
Coconut, unsweetened	25	3	8	1	–	1	92
Soy, unsweetened	52	1	40	8	–	4	92
Rice, unsweetened	35	1	62	6	–	0	92

FLAVORS

INGREDIENT	ENERGY (CAL)	FAT (G)	SODIUM (MG)	CARB (G)	FIBER (G)	PROTEIN (G)	WATER (%)
OILS & VINEGARS› 1 TBSP.							
Butter, unsalted	100	11	2	–	–	–	17
Coconut oil	116	14	–	–	–	–	–
Oils› canola, grapeseed, olive, truffle	124	14	–	–	–	–	–
Vinegar (apple cider, red wine)	3	–	1	–	–	–	99
Vinegar, balsamic	14	–	4	3	–	–	76

FLAVORS *(continued)*

INGREDIENT	ENERGY (CAL)	FAT (G)	SODIUM (MG)	CARB (G)	FIBER (G)	PROTEIN (G)	WATER (%)
CONDIMENTS & SWEETENERS› 2 TBSP.							
Applesauce, unsweetened	13	–	1	3	–	–	87
Barbeque sauce	53	–	392	13	–	–	60
Brown sugar	102	–	6	24	–	–	2
Chocolate chips, semisweet	140	8	–	20	2	2	18
Coconut milk, canned	210	21	30	5	–	2	86
Crystallized ginger› 1 tsp.	31	–	3	8	–	–	11
Honey› 1 tsp.	21	–	–	6	–	–	17
Jams (grape, raspberry, etc.)	102	–	12	28	–	–	31
Ketchup	30	–	334	8	–	–	69
Maple syrup	104	–	4	26	–	–	32
Molasses (unsulphured)	116	–	14	30	–	–	22
Preserves (cherry, blueberry, etc.)	70	–	50	18	–	–	35
Pumpkin butter	70	–	50	18	–	–	35
Soy sauce (low-sodium)	16	–	1,066	2	–	2	71
Sriracha sauce	30	–	600	6	–	–	80
Sugar (coarse/raw)	90	–	–	24	–	–	–
Tabasco› 1 tsp.	1	–	29	–	–	–	98
Vanilla extract› 1 tsp.	12	–	–	1	–	–	53
Vegetable bouillon› 1 cube (5 g)	15	1	840	–	–	–	4
SPICES› 1 TSP.							
Black pepper	5	–	1	1	1	–	10
Celery salt	–	–	1,160	–	–	–	–
Cinnamon	6	–	–	2	1	–	15
Curry powder	7	–	1	1	1	–	10
Garlic salt	–	–	1,960	–	–	–	–
Nutmeg	11	1	–	1	–	–	5
Salt	–	–	2,325	–	–	–	–

APPENDIX C
CONVERSIONS

COOKED & READY INGREDIENTS

If your recipe calls for cooked ingredients and you don't have them on hand, use the chart below to determine the uncooked quantities so you can prepare the ingredients for the recipe. Conversions are approximate and can vary depending on different varieties or brands.

INGREDIENT	UNCOOKED	COOKED
Bacon	8 oz.	¾–1 cup
Beans	1 cup	2–2½ cups
Chicken	8 oz.	1 cup
Grits	1 cup	3½–4 cups
Lentils	1 cup	2–2½ cups
Oats	1 cup	2 cups
Polenta	1 cup	3½ cups
Potatoes	8 oz.	1 cup
Quinoa	1 cup	4 cups
Rice, medium-grain	1 cup	2½–3 cups
Rice, short-grain	1 cup	2 cups

MEASUREMENT CONVERSIONS

VOLUME

U.S. STANDARD	
3 tsp. ↔ 1 tbsp.	
4 tbsp. ↔ ¼ cup	
8 tbsp. ↔ ½ cup	
16 tbsp. ↔ 1 cup	

IMPERIAL	
1 tbsp. ↔ ½ fl. oz.	
1 cup ↔ 8 fl. oz.	
1 cup ↔ ½ pint	
2 cups ↔ 1 pint	
4 cups ↔ 1 quart	
2 pints ↔ 1 quart	
4 quarts ↔ 1 gallon	

METRIC	
1 tsp. ↔ 5 ml	
1 tbsp. ↔ 15 ml	
¼ cup ↔ 60 ml	
½ cup ↔ 125 ml	
¾ cup ↔ 175 ml	
1 cup ↔ 250 ml	
1 pint ↔ 480 ml	
1 quart ↔ 1 liter	

WEIGHTS

METRIC	
1 oz. ↔ 30 grams	
2 oz. ↔ 60 grams	
4 oz. ↔ 115 grams	
8 oz. ↔ 225 grams	
1 pound ↔ 450 grams	
2 pounds ↔ 900 grams	

Note› Conversions have been rounded to make measuring easier.

INDEX

Note › t. indicates table; italic page numbers indicate pictures.

ACKNOWLEDGMENTS

BECAUSE THERE ARE always too many people to thank for their support and care, both in life and specifically on a project like this, I'd like to start by simply acknowledging anyone who had to work, deal, or talk to me in the last few months while finishing this book and letting you all know I'm sorry for my behavior. Thank you for not killing me or unfriending me on Facebook. As the age-old saying goes, "We keep our friends and family close by cooking for them but drive them away by writing about what we cook for them." Okay, I just made that up, but it's been an ironic pill to swallow in my recent experience, so I'm just saying.

I'm saying thanks to my mom, Almerick, Tonya, Dylan, and Madeline Lim. I promise that I'll never use the excuse "I can't. I'm working on the cookbook" ever again. Or at least not until Renee Jardine, the most wonderful editor in the world, cons me into writing a follow-up called *Still Hungry?* If that happens, you can blame her for both my angst and for how incredible this and any subsequent book will be.

Renee is as much responsible, if not entirely responsible, for making the *Feed Zone Cookbook* and *Portables* happen. She deserves a huge thank-you along with the incredible staff at VeloPress—Haley Berry, Vicki Hopewell, and Dave Trendler—and the talented photographers Jeanine Thurston and Caroline Treadway.

A special thanks also needs to be made to my incredible team at Skratch Labs for keeping me on track, holding down the fort, and actually letting me follow my bliss despite all of my ignorance. Remember these names: Aaron Foster, Ian MacGregor, Jen MacGregor, Jason Donald, Jon Robichaud, Jay Peery, Mary Kay Twargowski, Tadgh Parks, Lauren DeBell, Cole Kramer, Fika Otalora, and Casey Korbely—this book would not have happened without their commitment to Skratch or to making it from scratch.

And finally, where would I, or any of us, be without Chef Biju. Not only did he come over today to fix the leak on the top of the spout thing connected to my washing machine, he's taken everything I've ever learned and made it practical, teaching me things I didn't even know I didn't know. I know that sounds like magic and I know Biju would be the first to say that "it's just cooking." I'll be the first to say that Biju's cooking is magic. Thanks for the magic, Biju.

ALLEN LIM

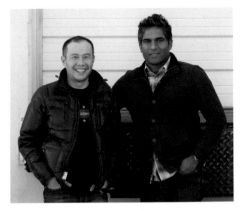

FIRST AND FOREMOST, I'd like to thank the dedicated staff at Velo-Press whose persistence and very, very long days made this book a reality: Renee Jardine, Haley Berry, Vicki Hopewell, Ted Costantino, and Dave Trendler.

I want to thank my family for teaching me a great love for food and the whole team at Skratch Labs for supporting Allen and me as we disappeared for weeks at a time to "research," cook, and write this book.

Thanks to all my friends and the amazing athletes who let me force-feed them random things while we worked out the ideas in this book: Taylor Phinney, Lucas Euser, Tim Johnson, Lynne Besette, Patrick Dempsey, Tom Boonen, Jens Voigt, Christian and Leah Vande Velde, Alex Howes, Peter Stetina, Craig Lewis, Julian Kyer, Evelyn Stevens, Jeremy Powers, Rebecca Rusch, Caiti Rowe, Rusty Perry, Spence Smith, Gus Flottman, Thomas Craven, Hincapie Sportswear Development Cycling Team, George Hincapie, Rich Hincapie, Tim Bauer, Todd Stockbauer, and David Shike.

I'm grateful to Connie Carpenter and Davis Phinney for the many hours spent driving and talking about life; to Jarka Duba, Chris Zenthoefer, Willie Ford, and Jon Robichaud for jumping into a very hot kitchen at Kona 2012; and to Khem and Molly for letting us take over their house for this photo shoot.

And of course thanks to my good friend Dr. Allen Lim, for continuing the ride, and for filling a book about cupcakes with delicious sciencey goodness that everyone can actually understand.

BIJU THOMAS

ABOUT THE AUTHORS

Born in the Philippines by way of China, **DR. ALLEN LIM** immigrated to the United States as a child with his parents, who were following the proverbial American dream.

While growing up in Los Angeles, Dr. Lim remembers being sucker-punched after participating in the annual Cinco de Mayo parade. He was caught between cultures—an angst that led him to ride his bicycle for hours at a time through the City of Angels. Those simple rides turned into a love affair with cycling that led him to study

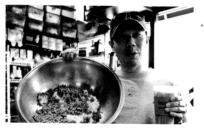

"ARMED WITH HIS RICE CAKE AND A PASSION FOR CYCLING, ALLEN LIM HAS CREATED A FOOD REVOLUTION IN THE PRO PELOTON."

CRAIG LEWIS *CHAMPION SYSTEMS PRO CYCLING TEAM*

the one subject that could improve his riding—exercise physiology. Dr. Lim eventually earned his PhD through the Department of Integrative Physiology at the University of Colorado at Boulder.

He began working on the pro cycling tour, hoping to use his knowledge to help others improve their riding. Lim's dream was nearly shattered by the rampant culture of doping he witnessed early in his career. He began working with a young TIAA-CREF cycling team to develop a method of testing for biological markers indicative of performance-enhancing drugs. Both the Garmin Professional Cycling Team and the Biological Passport were born out of this effort.

Continuing his fight for change, Dr. Lim started a company from scratch to bring healthy and authentic alternatives to the world of sports nutrition. With the success of *The Feed Zone Cookbook* and an all-natural sports drink from Skratch Labs, Dr. Lim finds himself still chasing something he fondly refers to as the American dream.

BIJU THOMAS IS A SELF-TAUGHT CHEF who moved with his family from Kerala, India, to Denver when he was 10. From his dad he learned that it's okay for men to cook, and from his mom he learned how to feed a lot of people quickly without breaking a sweat. He then learned from his four older brothers and younger sister that you should eat fast.

Biju has cooked with and for numerous cycling personalities, from Andy Hampsten and Davis Phinney to Jonathan Vaughters. While cooking for one of Vaughters's dinner parties, Biju met sports physiologist Dr. Allen Lim, who loved his light and flavorful approach to food.

Biju and Dr. Lim have worked with many of the world's top riders and cycling teams, from Lance Armstrong and Tom Boonen to the next generation of American stars on the rise. In

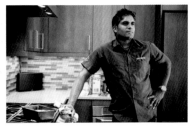

"BIJU HAS A WAY OF MAKING GREAT FOOD IN IMPOSSIBLE SITUATIONS. IT'S ALWAYS AN ADVENTURE WITH BIJU AT THE HELM."

JARKA DUBA *PRESIDENT POC USA*

2012, Biju was part of the team with Dr. Lim that launched the sports hydration company Skratch Labs in Boulder, Colorado.

During the 2013 cycling season, Biju will be chef to the BMC Racing Team, supporting Taylor Phinney, Tejay van Garderen, and Cadel Evans. He will also be chef to the Dempsey/Del Piero Racing team.

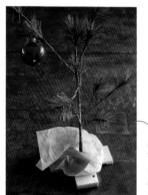

A special thank-you to Ben, Ella, Molly, and Khemarin for their generosity in allowing us to shoot in their beautiful home during the holidays.

Art direction, design, and composition by **Vicki Hopewell**

Cover design by **Andy Omel**

Recipe photography by **Jeanine Thurston Photography**

Photography of the cooking process and Skratch Labs summer training camp by **Caroline Treadway,** with color correction by **Jackie Donnelly Baisa**

Additional photography› Tim De Waele: pp. 4, 22 ★ Jamie Kripke: pp. 19, 48, 59 ★ Lauren DeBell: p. 269

Photographs for athlete profiles› Graham Watson: pp. xii, 155 ★ © Red Bull Media House: p. xiv ★ Brian Hodes: pp. xv, 198 ★ John Dickey: p. 78 ★ CJFoto.com: p. 85 ★ Brad Kaminski: p. 99 ★ Todd Meier Photography: p. 126 ★ Casey B. Gibson: p. 173 ★ Timothy Carlson: p. 187 ★ Nils Nilsen: pp. 218–219 ★ AP Images/Sergey Ponomarev: p. 234 ★ Tim Kemple: p. 246

Photo shoot locations courtesy of the **Seng/Ware family** and **Aaron Foster**

Nutrition analysis by **Jessie Shafer**

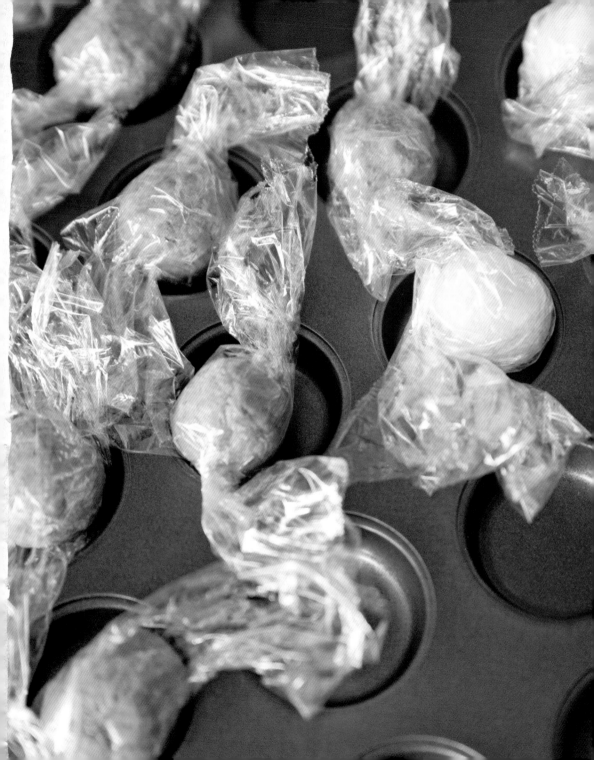

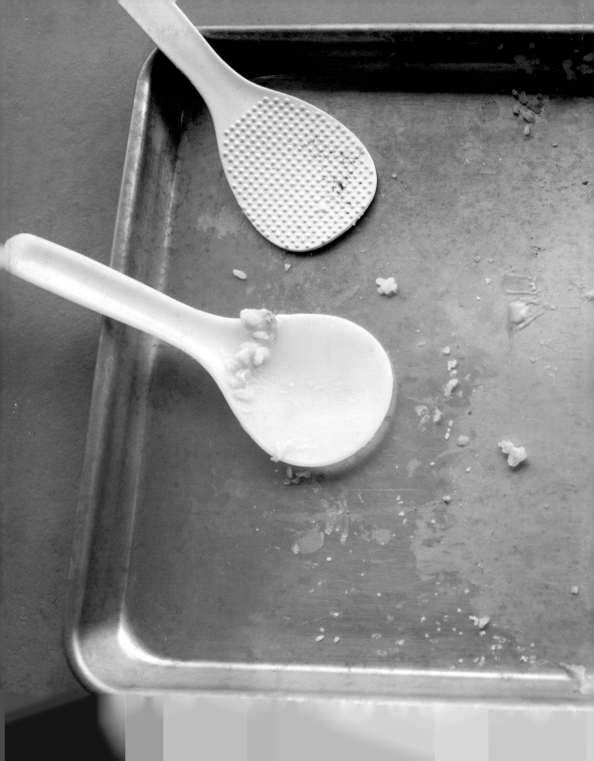